A REVOLUTIONARY APPROACH TO PROSTATE CANCER
A Physician and Patient Perspective

Drs. Aubrey Pilgrim and E. David Crawford

Articles and Chapters by over 20 Other Doctors and Survivors

eShore

Pittsburgh, PA

ISBN 1-58501-015-4

Trade Paperback
©Copyright 2002
Dr. Aubrey Pilgrim and Dr. E. David Crawford
All rights reserved
First Printing—2002
Library of Congress #2001090118

Request for information should be addressed to:

CeShore Publishing Company
The Sterling Building
440 Friday Road
Pittsburgh, PA 15209
www.ceshore.com

CeShore is an imprint of SterlingHouse Publisher, Inc.
Cover Design: Michelle S. Lenkner—SterlingHouse Publisher
Page Design: Bernadette Kazmarski

This publication includes images from Corel Draw 8 which are
protected by the copyright laws of the U.S., Canada and elsewhere.

Printed in the United States of America

ACKNOWLEDGEMENT

There are several abstracts reprinted throughout this book to illustrate studies and research. We want to thank all those people who did the studies and research.

There are also many doctors and patients who contributed to this book. We wish to thank them all for helping us all to better understand this beast.

We also want to thank Susan Shepard for helping to proofread and edit this book.

DEDICATION

We wrote about Russ Ingram, Len Snyder, Scott Barker, Ed Piepmeier, Lloyd Ney, Jerry Man and several others in the original edition of this book. We are sad to tell you that they lost the battle. Thousands of others died this year, last year and each year in the past. Over 400,000 men have died from prostate cancer in the U.S. during the last ten years. We dedicate this book to the memory of all those men.

TABLE OF CONTENTS

FOREWORD

Dear Reader;

If you have just been diagnosed with prostate cancer (PCa), and you don't have a computer with a modem, then you should go out and buy one now. Even if you have to skip the rent, or put off buying your kids a new pair of $100 sneakers, or you have to eat beans for a while, buy a computer and get online. One of the best ways to defeat prostate cancer is to be informed. One of the best ways to be informed is to be on the Internet.

There are several on-line sites that can help you decide what treatment to choose. The Prostate-Help Mailing List (PHML) and the Prostate Problems Mailing List (PPML) are both free. There are several medical doctors that answer posted questions. There are also many, many first hand reports and accounts from patients who have experienced the various treatments. One of the best is the Prostate-Help Mailing List (PHML). To subscribe send e-mail to:

> listserv@home.ease.lsoft.com
> Subject: leave blank
> Message: subscribe prostate-help

To subscribe to the PPML, send an email to:

> LISTSERV@listserv.acor.org
> Subject: (blank or a dash)
> Message: subscribe prostate yourfirstname yourlastname

The PHML and the PPML are *very* active lists, generating upwards of 100K on a typical day. That is why you need a fast modem and a large hard disk.

SeedPods is a mailing list for those interested in brachytherapy (radioactive seed implants) as a treatment for prostate cancer. To subscribe, send an email:

> To: majordomo@prostatepointers.org
> Subject: (blank or a dash)
> Message: subscribe seedpods

There are several other important web sites listed in the chapter on Resources. I have included a few accounts that were posted by PCa survivors on PHML and PPML in this book.

You don't have to have the most powerful and biggest computer available. But get one with a large hard disk, about 10 gigabytes and the fastest modem available. The 56Kb modems are the fastest used on the Internet at the moment.

The net proceeds from the sale of this book are being donated to the US TOO International Support Group organization. Call them at 1-800-808-7866 and have them put you on their mailing list.

This book would not have been possible without the help and input of the several doctors listed as coauthors and the many contributions from prostate cancer survivors.

We believe that everything stated in this book is true. But what is true today may not be true tomorrow. One of the first things that you learn in science, and especially about prostate cancer, is that there are few absolutes. In this book we make very few statements that are absolute.

> *We wish you all the very best—*
> *Drs. Aubrey Pilgrim and David Crawford*

FOREWORD FROM US TOO

Aubrey Pilgrim is an unusually talented man and Dr. David Crawford is a giant among urologists; teaming up for this new publication generates a book that is absolutely jammed with up to date information as well as much of the "how to" that makes coping with prostate cancer a more facile undertaking. Because so much of the advice and scientific approach fit in with US TOO we are pleased to recommend this book.

US TOO was founded in 1990 at the University of Chicago urology offices where five survivors talking together in the waiting room decided it was helpful to share experiences. In mentioning this to the doctors, the M.D.'s agreed to invite their patients to an initial meeting held early in February. These men went on to spread the word and by the fall of 1993 when a new board was elected incorporating the original founders, US TOO had expanded to over 50 chapters.

The ensuing six and a half years have been exciting ones. US TOO now has 350 very active prostate cancer support chapters as well as another 150 chapters that are considered satellite chapters. As we meet together to support one another, specialists in each chapter step forward with the latest information obtained from journals, newspapers or other media and a number of men work tirelessly each day to bring late breaking news from the Internet. US TOO has grown to be the largest prostate cancer support organization because of the volunteer members who pull together for the common good and for the support of one another.

Newly diagnosed men picking up this book will receive the same unselfish, freely given support and data as all of us have received from our predecessors. You in turn will find the great satisfaction we have found in helping other men who come after you. Prostate cancer is often an aggressive disease but we have to live with and try to maintain a substantial quality of life.

US TOO has received wonderful cooperation and support from prostate cancer survivors, their families, the medical profession and many government entities.

We are especially indebted to the authors in dedicating proceeds of this book to support US TOO programs which are run by volunteers with a sprinkling of the necessary supervisory paid individuals.

This gives us a use of funds of about 93% direct support with only 7% for ancillary services. But we never have enough money to do all that we would like to do. US TOO is a tax deductible organization.

Some day prostate cancer will be conquered; in the meantime, we live with it and are much better for continuing our support of one another and contributing to the support of scientists as they move forward with novel new approaches in disease control.

US TOO welcomes your questions, your support, your need for information and just plain straight talk. Please call us for the location of a support group near you. All of us volunteers look forward each day to the opportunity of helping new people through the tough beginning stages of prostate cancer and continuing the fight to eventually lick the disease.

> *Best regards,*
> *Henry A. Porterfield*
> *Chairman/CEO US TOO International*
> *930 North York Rd., Suite 50*
> *Hinsdale, IL 60521-2993*
> *Phone 630-323-1002 800-808-7866*
> *www.ustoo.com*

The Latest Treatment Options For Prostate Cancer

INTRODUCTION

Drs. E. David Crawford & Aubrey Pilgrim

THE PURPOSE OF THIS BOOK

The primary purpose of this book is to help inform you of your treatment options for prostate cancer. Many men panic when they hear the word cancer and just want it out. Please do not panic. It is not a death sentence. Before you do anything, you should know about all of your options. You can then choose a treatment that is best for you. It is your body, your disease and your responsibility to make an informed choice of treatment.

The treatment options are discussed in separate chapters in this book. Most of these chapters were written by doctors who specialize in that particular therapy. However, we have to tell you that each one of these doctors is biased. They believe that their protocol and therapy is the best. If they didn't believe this, then they should not be practicing that specialty. So don't be surprised if a surgeon tells you that surgery is the best option. Or a radiologist says that radiation is best, or a brachytherapist says that seed implants are best.

There may be cases where one or the other of these therapies may be best for you. You should be aware that there may be no best treatment. A prostate cancer treatment that is optimal for one person may not be best for another. We are all different and there are different types and stages of prostate cancer. For some, the outcome may be the same, no matter which therapy is chosen.

We also have to tell you that no matter what treatment option you choose, there will be complications. Some may be minor, some may be rather drastic. But you have to remember that you have cancer. Your life is going to be changed. You will have to learn to make compromises and perhaps a few sacrifices.

We can't possibly begin to tell you all you need to know in this book. Besides, there are new developments and new treatments being introduced every day. In order to learn all you can and keep up to date, you need a computer so that you can access the Internet and the tremendous amount of information there. There are several search engines such as www.yahoo.com, www.excite.com, www.lycos.com and others, which can search the millions of articles and information on the Internet in just seconds. It is a fantastic resource. Computers are fairly inexpensive now. You don't need the fastest, most powerful top of the line for accessing the Internet.

You will probably be running into a lot of unfamiliar medical terms. We have included a glossary in the appendix, but it cannot possibly list all the terms that you may need to know. We suggest that you invest in a medical dictionary such as Taber's Cyclopedic Medical Dictionary. It is fairly small and has a wealth of information. Another book that might be helpful is the Appleton & Langes Drug Guide. It lists and describes most of the current drugs. If you have a computer to access the Internet, you can order these books and many others from www.amazon.com or www.barnesandnoble.com.

The prostate gland is a small structure about the size of a walnut. It encircles the urethra just below the bladder. The prostate gland is a part of the reproductive system. It provides the major part of the fluid that is mixed with the sperm cells as they are ejaculated.

Many men are not even aware that they have a prostate gland and it may never cause them any problems. Even though small, it kills 30,000 to 40,000 men each year in the U.S.

One third of the men in this country over 50 years old have prostate cancer. If you are over 50 years old and in a room with two other men over 50, one of you has prostate cancer. Men in battle always think that it is the other man who is going to be killed. So we always believe that it is the other person who has the cancer. But it doesn't always happen that way. However, before you panic, you should know that many of those prostate cancers are latent and will never cause any harm. Yet prostate cancer kills more men than any other cancer except for lung cancer.

We know that a person's lifestyle can contribute to cancer. We know that everyone should get a bit of exercise now and then and enjoy life. Being unhappy can definitely alter your immune system. Being happy or unhappy is often one's choice.

There are hundreds of preventive measures that you can take that can help prevent you from getting cancer. The odds will be on your side if you follow all of the common sense rules for prevention. But there is no guarantee that you can prevent it. Here is a rule that will be repeated several times in this book:

The first rule when it comes to cancer is that there are no rules!

WHAT'S IN THIS BOOK

You will need to understand a bit about cancer in general so we talk about cancer in Chapter One. In later chapters we will discuss the prostate and the rest of the body. There will be chapters on each of the major treatment options. We will talk about the various methods of diagnosis and treatments and side effects. We will have photos and drawings of the prostate. And we will list several resources and support groups that can help you. We will even include a bit of humor now and then.

Some who are reading this book may already know a lot about these subjects. Others may know very little. We will try to take the middle ground and try to explain the subjects so that every one will understand.

The net proceeds from the sale of this book are being donated to the US TOO International Support Group organization. Call them at 1-800-808-7866 and have them put you on their mailing list.

This book would not have been possible without the help and input of the several doctors listed as co-authors and the many contributions from prostate cancer survivors.

We believe that everything stated in this book is true. But what is true today may not be true tomorrow. One of the first things that you learn in science, and especially about prostate cancer, is that there are few absolutes. In this book we make very few statements that are absolute, except for this statement:

The answer to cancer is early detection.

Chapter One
AN OVERVIEW
Drs. Aubrey Pilgrim and E. David Crawford

TREATMENT OPTIONS

If you have been diagnosed with prostate cancer, you will have several treatment options. The doctor has several tools to help make the diagnosis, such as a digital rectal exam, the PSA blood test, ultrasound images and several other tests. These tests and his expertise will help to assign a clinical stage (CS) to the cancer. The diagnosis may help you determine what treatment to choose.

Treatments that you may consider include watchful waiting, surgery or radical prostatectomy, radiation, including external beam and seed implants, cryosurgery, hormones and chemotherapy. Depending on several factors, combinations of the treatments may be necessary. For instance, external beam radiation or hormone treatments may be added or combined with any of the primary treatments. Your doctor may recommend the treatment, but it is your body and it is your choice as to what treatment you want. It should be an informed choice. This book can help you make an informed choice.

You could choose any of these treatments. But depending on your age, health and life expectancy, some treatments may be preferable to the others. Other factors that may influence your decision is the PSA number and the Gleason score.

Those men whose prostate cancer is detected before it has a chance to escape the prostate gland capsule have more treatment choices. They can be treated and usually cured. But once the cancer has escaped the prostate and become advanced, it can be treated, but may not be cured.

WATCHFUL WAITING

An older person with a fairly short life expectancy might choose Watchful Waiting. This might be a good choice for anyone with a low PSA and low grade tumor. The PSA level would be often checked and if it appeared that the cancer was changing, then other treatment could be chosen. Remember that watchful waiting is taking the chance that you will die of something else other than prostate cancer. Most cancers will progress, but at different rates.

RADICAL PROSTATECTOMY

A radical prostatectomy is the "gold standard" and is performed more often than any other procedure. If the cancer is still confined to the prostate, a radical prostatectomy would completely remove all of the cancer cells. Usually, a radical prostatectomy is recommended for younger men in their late forties or fifties, who have a fairly long life expectancy.

A disadvantage is that a radical prostatectomy is a major operation. A small percentage of men are left with incontinence and many have impotence problems or erectile dysfunction (ED). And even with the most expert surgeon, there is a chance that some of the cancer cells may have already escaped and the cancer may recur. After a radical prostatectomy, the PSA should be undetectable. If it is detected it would indicate that the cancer has recurred.

In some cases, radiation may be used in addition to the surgery. Hormone therapy may also be used before and after surgery.

RADIATION

Radiation is usually not as traumatic as surgery. Some data for radiation seems to indicate that it may be equivalent to surgery or any of the other treatments. If you are an older man you might choose some form of radiation. This might also be a better choice for a person in poor health who might not be able to withstand the trauma of a major operation such as a radical prostatectomy. There may be a lesser incidence of incontinence and impotence with radiation. However both of these can occur with this treatment.

One disadvantage is that radiation may not kill all of the cancer cells. If any are left behind, the cancer may recur. If you are fairly old, leaving a few cells may not be that bad. It may take ten to twenty years for a cancer to become significant. If your life expectancy is less than that, why worry?

There are several different types of radiation such as conventional x-rays, 3D conformal, Proton Beam, and seed implants. Brachytherapy, or seed implants, is the placement of radioactive "seeds", about the size of a small grain of rice, in the prostate. We only have data for seed implant treatment over the last 12 years. It appears to be as effective as any of the other treatments with less side effects. However, the jury is still out on its long term cure rates.

If the cancer recurs and the PSA rises after radiation, hormone therapy may be instituted.

CRYOSURGERY

Cryosurgery uses probes inserted into the prostate to freeze the cancer cells. It is also fairly new. It has some promising results over the last ten years, but it does have some undesirable side effects such as impotence.

If the PSA rises after cryosurgery, hormone therapy or radiation may be necessary.

HORMONES

At one time hormone therapy was reserved almost exclusively for advanced cancers. Now many men with localized, low grade cancer are being treated with hormones. The antiandrogen monotherapy is one of the least invasive of all treatments. This drug treatment can often stop the tumor growth in the less aggressive type cancers.

If there is an indication that the cancer has advanced beyond the prostate or metastasized, hormone therapy would be the treatment choice. Prostate cancer cells thrive on testosterone from the testicles and androgenic hormones from the adrenal glands. The cancer progression can be slowed or stopped by preventing or blocking the production of these hormones. One way to block the testosterone is to have an orchiectomy, a nice way of saying castration. There are certain drugs that can block the production of testosterone just as if one has been castrated. There are also synthetic drugs such as Casodex and Flutamide that mimic the adrenal androgens. If the receptors of the cancer cells accept these synthetic drugs, then the actual androgens are blocked.

One disadvantage of castration and hormone therapy is that it can completely eliminate the libido and the person may lose all interest in sex. He may also have hot flashes, his breasts may become enlarged (gynecomastia), and he may feel tired and weak. However, considering that metastatic cancer can kill, most men will gladly suffer the side effects of hormone therapy.

CHEMOTHERAPY

In some men the combined hormone therapy (CHT) may only work for a few years before the cancer cells become refractory, that is, they learn to live without the hormones. When this happens, there are other drugs and chemotherapies that can be instituted.

Chemotherapy is usually reserved for the treatment of last resort. Although, a number of new regimens have been developed which offer new hope in controlling the disease. Because of these promising results, chemotherapy is being used earlier in the disease.

Dr. Maha Hussain, an oncologist, recommends that it be used early instead of using it as a last resort. She rationalizes that the chemotherapy may inhibit or prevent many of the hormone independent cells from proliferating.

TRYING TO IDENTIFY THE KILLERS

There are several tests that can help try to determine which cancers are killers and which are harmless. One important test is to make a PSA chart to see if there are any active changes. If the PSA number begins to go up, then it may indicate that the cancer is growing. The normal PSA for a man in his 50s may be 0 to 4 nanograms per milliliter (ng/ml); for a 70-year-old man a PSA of 5 ng/ml may be normal. Some men who have computers have used spreadsheet programs to track their PSA and history.

Generally, for those men who have a significant cancer that is still confined to the prostate, the PSA may be 2.5 to 20 ng/ml. However, the risk of spread outside the prostate may be nearly 50% if the PSA is greater than 10ng/ml. If the cancer has metastasized, the PSA may be from 20 ng/ml up to 6000 ng/ml or more.

Ordinarily, since each cancer cell produces a finite amount of PSA, the amount of PSA is a fairly good indication of how much cancer is present. But remember, the first rule is that there are no rules when it comes to cancer.

A friend has a PSA of 50, yet they had to do several biopsies before they found a small cancer. A biopsy or small sample of the prostate cells can also indicate how serious the cancer is. A pathologist can look at the cells and assign a Gleason grade to them. Dr. Gleason determined that there were five different grades of cancer as the cells mutated from normal to very abnormal. (More about Gleason grades in Chapter 5). With a PSA of 50, you would expect to find a fairly high Gleason score of six or seven. His was 3.

Some men may have very aggressive life-threatening cancer but the PSA may be very low. It could be that the cancer cells have mutated to the point where they can no longer produce PSA.

DIGITAL RECTAL EXAMINATIONS

Digital Rectal Examinations (DRE) and ultrasound can also be used to periodically check for changes. The doctor may be able to feel any new growth or lumps in the prostate. Any such findings could indicate an aggressive cancer.

METASTASIS

If the cancer has metastasized, it often starts new colonies of prostate cancer in other parts of the body and often in the bones. A bone scan can identify these colonies in the bones. They can be seen as "hot spots" on special x-rays.

ProstaScint is a fairly new test that uses monoclonal antibodies that are specific for prostate cells. The antibodies are tagged with a radioactive material and then injected into the body. The antibodies will seek out and accumulate in prostate tissues. A scanning device can then locate the radioactive cells. If there is an accumulation of cells outside the prostate, then you know that there is metastasis.

AFTER-EFFECTS OF TREATMENT

When discovered before it metastasizes to the rest of the body, the cancer can usually be successfully treated. Even if it has metastasized, you can still be treated and your life can usually be extended. However, you should know that for most treatments there will be some side effects. After the treatments your life will be changed forever to some degree. Depending on the treatment, you may have some degree of incontinence.

You may or may not be able to achieve an erection. If you have a radical prostatectomy, you will never be able to ejaculate again. Orgasms and ejaculation are two separate things. If you could have orgasms before the operation, you will still be able to have orgasms after. It won't be quite the same, but you will still be alive and can expect to live a fairly normal lifespan. You might even live longer than a person who has never had prostate cancer because you may wake up and start taking better care of yourself.

EDUCATE YOURSELF

There are a few doctors who recommend that the prostate should be removed or irradiated, no matter what the stage or significance. For some patients, the cancer may not be a threat. Unfortunately, we have no absolute way to determine which cancers are insignificant and which are the ones that can kill you. There are some statistics that can help such as the Partin Tables and the Artificial Neural Network (ANN). They will be discussed in Chapter 6. By studying these tables and statistics you can get a fairly good idea of what kind of treatment you should have.

For those men whose cancer has metastasized and escaped the prostate, removal of the prostate may not help them. However, some doctors do remove the prostate even when metastasis is evident. They do this to debulk the tumor and ease the burden on the body. Not everyone agrees that this is helpful.

Usually if there is evidence of metastases, the men may be treated with drugs, radiation, chemotherapy, hormones or by castration. Even if there is widespread metastases, with proper treatments, many men are able to live for several years. If some other disease does not kill the man, eventually the metastatic cancer will. At the present time we have few cures for any kind of cancer that has metastasized whether it is prostate, breast, colon, lung or whatever. We can only try to slow the growth of the cancer and alleviate any pain. This does not mean that anyone should give up hope. With proper treatment and care, many men survive as long as those without cancer.

PROSTATE CANCER NOW NUMBER ONE

About 180,000 men were diagnosed with prostate cancer this year. It has now surpassed lung cancer as the number one diagnosed cancer in men. Lung cancer is still the number one killer. Counting men and women, lung cancer kills about 150,000 people each year. Prostate cancer kills between 30,000 and 40,000 men each year.

One reason that prostate cancer is now the number one diagnosed cancer is because more and more men are being checked for prostate cancer. The simple prostate specific antigen (PSA) blood test and ultrasound, added to the standard digital rectal exam (DRE), makes it much easier to detect prostate cancer while it is still in the early stages.

If a man gets lung cancer because he smokes, he usually has no one to blame but himself. But if he gets prostate cancer it may not be his fault. We don't know exactly what causes it. If a man lives past 80 years old, there is about an 80 percent chance that he will have prostate cancer to some degree. At this age though, he will probably die of some other cause before the prostate cancer kills him. If he lives to be 100 years old, the chances that he has prostate cancer is about 100 percent.

Dr. Linus Pauling was diagnosed with prostate cancer at 92 years old. A reporter asked him why his Vitamin C intake did not protect him. He said, "Had I not been taking Vitamin C, I might have got prostate cancer 40 years ago." Dr. Pauling died from prostate cancer a little over a year later at 93 years old. Dr. Pauling was the only person who ever received two Nobel prizes in his own name, one for chemistry and one for peace.

From autopsies done on young men 20 to 30 years old who died in accidents, war or other causes, about 30% of them have a small beginning prostate cancer tumor. About 38% of those who were 30 to 40 at the time of death had small cancerous tumors. Most of those cancers would have never been a threat. The challenge is trying to detect and treat the bad ones.

SYMPTOMS

There may be no symptoms. Dr. Robert Kelly, a medical doctor in his early 50s belongs to one of our local prostate cancer support groups in the Los Angeles area. He had no symptoms when his prostate cancer was first detected. It had spread throughout his body. A normal PSA for a man his age should be less than 4 ng/ml. His PSA was over 524 ng/ml. He has had several hormonal and chemotherapy treatments and is still doing well 9 years later.

Here are a few symptoms that you may experience:

A small urine stream, hesitancy, having to go a lot during the day, having to get up several times at night, any kind of pain in your back or pelvic area.

Almost everybody has back pain now and then due to straining a muscle or other injury. If the cancer escapes the prostate gland, it often invades the bones of the spine or the pelvis. It may cause severe pain that is quite different than the pain from a strained muscle.

Again, and again, there are no rules, so you may have no symptoms. Prostate cancer can truly be a silent killer.

SECOND OPINIONS

If you have had a PSA test and a biopsy that clearly shows cancer, it may not be much help to get a second opinion. It will probably be the same as the first one. Even if you get a third or fourth opinion, it may still be about the same as the first one, but do it anyway. It may help you make a better decision as to your treatment. If you don't make an effort to learn all you can before making a decision, you may later feel that it wasn't the best decision. Remember that you will have to live with whatever treatment decision you make for the rest of your life. It should be an informed decision.

Be aware that if you ask several doctors as to what treatment you should have, you may get several different opinions.

It may be in your best interests to get a second opinion from a Cancer Center where a multidisciplinary team will evaluate your disease. Many such centers have a second opinion clinic which is staffed by specialist in the fields of Urology, Radiation Oncology, and Medical Oncology. Take your time. Remember that most prostate cancers grow slowly. It may have taken 10 years or more for your prostate cancer to have become clinically evident so you are not going to die overnight.

In most cases you can wait a couple of months or more, depending on your PSA, your Gleason score, your age, and several other factors, before making such an important decision.

CHOOSE THE BEST DOCTOR

If you must have surgery, technically, any medical doctor could operate on you. But you want an experienced urological surgeon. Try to make sure that you have the best doctor. Talk to some of his patients, nurses, and other doctors. Find out how many operations he has performed. Usually, the more procedures a doctor has performed, the more skilled he or she is.

Even if it costs you extra to get a better and more experienced doctor, remember that it is only money. If you don't take the time to find a good doctor, you may regret it the rest of your life. Your quality of life may be diminished for the rest of your life.

Money becomes quite insignificant when you consider the consequences. If you don't have the money, then explore every way possible of getting the treatment your life deserves. Join a support group. Buy a computer and go on-line. Try the community services and hospitals. Contact the American Cancer Society for help.

No matter what treatment you choose, do your homework. Find out all you can about the doctor. Talk to his patients and anyone else who knows him. Don't be embarrassed, or afraid that you will hurt the doctor's feelings. After all, it is your life and the quality of your life for the rest of your life, that is at stake.

FACING THE INEVITABLE

Something that we may not like to confront is a discussion of end of life decisions. We never know when our time will come. Many hospitals now provide an "advanced directive" or "living will" for the patient to sign. California and many other states have a "Durable Power of Attorney." Among other things, it allows you to name a relative or friend to act and make medical decisions in your behalf if you become unable to do so. In the vast majority of cases, these papers will not be needed, but just in case, signing the paper could save a lot of problems for your loved ones.

BEWARE OF QUACKERY

If you have been diagnosed with prostate cancer, you may panic and start reaching out for any kind of treatment or drug that might help you. There is no need to panic and rush into anything. You have time to make the best decisions.

There are many charlatans, quacks and absolutely unscrupulous and dishonest people who will try to get their hands in your pockets. They have no morals or any conscience. They prey on sick people and will take advantage of you and your condition if you let them. There are many men whose cancer is no longer responding to treatments. These men may reach out for any hope, for anything at all that might help them. No one can blame them for trying. But we can blame the charlatans and quacks who knowingly offer them false hope.

MEDICAL MIRANDA

Dr. Stephen Strum is a medical oncologistand founder of the Prostate Cancer Research Institute. He specializes in prostate cancer treatments. He developed a Medical Miranda, such as the one read to criminal suspects when they are arrested. His Medical Miranda says:

> "You have the right to know your diagnosis,
>
> You have the right to understand the principles of evaluation and treatment,
>
> You have the right to be familiar with the pros and cons of available treatment options."

There is at least one other right that we would add:

> "You have the right to choose whatever treatment you want."

There are a large number of different treatments and methods of treatments for prostate cancer. The treatment that you receive will be your choice. Most doctors will make a recommendation for treatment, but the ultimate choice will be yours to make. Most of the major treatment options are quite similar in outcomes.

Unfortunately, if your cancer was not discovered before it metastasized, your choices of treatment may be limited.

The answer to cancer is early detection.

Chapter Two
WHAT CANCER IS
Drs. Aubrey Pilgrim, E. David Crawford

and Several Contributors

Cancer is one of the most fearsome words in our language. Some people equate it to a death sentence, but many cancer patients live longer than those who have never had cancer. One reason is that they begin to start taking better care of themselves. If discovered in time, many cancers can be cured or treated so that the person can live a fairly normal and extended life.

Each year, over 1,500,000 people are diagnosed with some type of cancer. One out of every two men and one out of every three women will be diagnosed with some type of cancer in their lifetime. About 80 percent of these cancers are preventable because they are due to four major factors:

Lifestyle, which includes smoking, diet and infectious agents;

Workplace, which includes chemicals, fibers and radiation;

General Environmental contaminants in air, water and food;

Clinical and other medications and radiation.

All these factors combine with the age of the patients, gender, ethnicity, genetics, nutrition, immune function and any preexisting disease to cause cancer.

Frederica P. Perea wrote an article for the May 1996 issue of Scientific American Magazine titled Uncovering New Clues to Cancer Risk. The investigator says that there are over 400 chemicals that have been shown to be carcinogenic in humans and animals. Many of these carcinogens are in our air, water, food supplies and the workplace. If we could eliminate environmental exposures, it is estimated that cancer incidence could be reduced by 90 percent.

The deaths of most of those 560,000 people, who die each year due to all types of cancer, could be prevented if the cancer is detected early. **The answer to cancer is early detection.**

THE MOST COMMON CANCERS

Skin cancer is the number one diagnosed cancer, but it is fairly easy to treat and does not kill many people. Lung cancer is still the number one killer of men and women. It kills about 150,000 men and women each year. There are about 180,000 cases of prostate cancer diagnosed each year and it kills 30,000 to 40,000 men each year. Breast cancer is the fourth most diagnosed cancer with about 180,000 detected each year. About 43,000 women die from it each year.

Just a few years ago, there were more incidences of diagnosed breast cancer than prostate cancer. But more men are now being made aware of prostate cancer and are concerned enough to get a check up. However there are still a large number of men who have the disease and are not aware of it. At least one man out of every ten over 50 has prostate cancer. For black men, the risk is even higher. One out of every eight black men over 50 will have prostate cancer. At this time, there are about 40 million men in the U.S. over 50. This means that there are over four million men with prostate cancer. For many of these men, the cancer will never become significant.

Before 1990, the incidence of diagnosed prostate cancer was about half what it is today. Even the number of men who died from it was less. Before 1985, the primary method of prostate cancer diagnosis was by digital rectal exam (DRE). This is the test that the doctor does when he has you bend over and he or she puts his gloved finger in your rectum. The prostate can be felt through the rectal wall. About 70% of all prostate cancer is the area that can be felt through the rectal wall.

Today we have the prostate specific antigen (PSA) blood test which is much more accurate in detecting prostate cancer, so many more cases are being diagnosed. One reason more men are dying from prostate cancer today, in spite of the early diagnosis, is because fewer men are dying from heart disease, lung cancer and other diseases. Many men are now living long enough for their prostate cancer to kill them.

We don't know how to prevent cancers, but most of them can be easily cured if they are discovered early. Usually a breast cancer or prostate cancer that is found early is fairly inexpensive to treat and cure. However, if the cancer is advanced when first detected, it can be treated, but it is incurable. It is also very expensive to treat. Doctors can offer palliative treatments to ease the pain and to try to keep the patient as comfortable as possible. In many cases, even with metastatic cancer, the patient can live a fairly good life. Of course the quality of life can never be the same. We will say it again and again, the best way to fight cancer is an early checkup and early detection.

FAMILY RISKS

We have known for some time that there is a definite familial risk among close male family members for prostate cancer. Some studies have indicated that close female relatives of men who have prostate cancer have a higher risk of getting breast cancer. It works both ways so male relatives of women who have breast cancer have a 40% to 50% higher risk of prostate cancer.

Men over 40 should have a prostate checkup at least once a year. Women over 40 should have a breast cancer checkup at least once a year.

CANCER TERMS

There are several terms that you may not be familiar with. We have a comprehensive glossary in the Appendix. Here are a few of the common terms that we will be discussing in this chapter.

Cancer

Cancer is the abnormal and uncontrolled growth of some of the cells in a body. About 90% of cancers are called carcinomas. Some of the others are called sarcomas, which are usually found in connective tissues; osteomas, or bone cancer; melanomas, or cancers from moles. Cancer is from Greek which means crab.

Tumor

Tumor is Latin, meaning a swelling. The—*oma* in carcinoma is a Greek suffix that means tumor. So cancers may also be called tumors, but not all tumors are cancerous. Some tumors are benign growths or lumps that may not be life threatening.

We want to stress the fact that **the first rule about cancer is that there are no rules**. Quite often, but not always, the cancer will be a hard lump. Ordinary cells usually have spaces between them filled with lymphatic fluid and the tissue is rather soft. Many cancers are hard lumps because the cells are packed very close together. A cancer tumor may have ten times more cells than an equivalent amount of normal tissue.

A tumor may also be called a neoplasm. *Neo* is Greek for new and *plasma* is Latin for form or mold. A neoplasm has come to mean a new and abnormal formation of tissue.

The term carcinoma is derived from the Greek *karkinos* which means crab. The ancient physicians of the Hippocratic school thought that the cancer they saw in their patients looked like a many legged crab. The grasping branches of the cancer that spread out reminded them of the claws on the crab.

Cancer is like a parasite. A parasite is an organism that lives within or upon a host. It contributes nothing to the benefit, welfare or survival of the host. Parasites may be such organisms as fleas, lice, tapeworms, fungi, bacteria, and viruses. Often the parasites will become so greedy that they will suck the life right out of the host. Cancer can do the same.

Metastasis

Metastasis is from Greek—*meta* means after, beyond, or over—*stasis* means to stand—so metastasis means to stand beyond or over.

As long as a cancer remains encapsulated as a tumor, it may not be much of a problem, unless it is growing on or in a vital organ such as the brain. But it becomes an incurable problem when the cells begin to spread and metastasize. The cancer may send out fingers and invade nearby tissues. Normal tissue does not invade neighboring tissues.

A few cells may break away and escape in the blood stream. These cells may then set up a distant colony. If the cells came from the prostate, then it will still be prostate cancer even if it is located in distant areas of the body such as the lymph nodes or the bones of the spine.

Digital Rectal Exam (DRE)

Part of the prostate can be readily felt through the rectum. An experienced doctor can do a digital rectal exam (DRE) and determine if there is any unusual growth or abnormality. A normal prostate is fairly soft and uniform. If there is prostate cancer present, depending on the stage and location, it may be hard or indurated, which means hardened. It may have lumps and nodules. If there seems to be any abnormality, the doctor may have a PSA test done, then perhaps ultrasound tests and a biopsy.

A DRE and a PSA test can detect most all prostate cancer. Most prostate cancers are slow growing and may not cause any problem as long as they remain encapsulated in the prostate. If they live to an old age, most all men will die with prostate cancer, but not necessarily because of it. It has been estimated that 80 percent of 80-year-old men have prostate cancer to some degree. If a man lives to be 100 years old, the chances are about 100 percent that he will have prostate cancer to some degree. Many of the cancers found in these cases may still be contained within the prostate capsule and have not caused any problems.

Prostate Specific Antigen (PSA)

It is difficult to think of anyone having cancer as being fortunate. But prostate cancer patients may be considered fortunate in that the cancer creates a substance that can be readily detected. The prostate produces Prostate Specific Antigen (PSA) that is present in the blood stream. If cancer is present, the amount of PSA will usually be elevated. Quite often the amount of PSA in the blood will correspond roughly with the amount and size of the tumor. Usually the more tumor cells, the more PSA is present. A blood test for PSA may cost less than $50, which is very inexpensive when you consider that it could save a person's life.

Once the prostate has been removed there should be no PSA in the patient's blood. If PSA is still being produced then we know that the operation was not done soon enough to prevent metastasis. Cancer that has metastasized to some other part of the body may be treatable but not curable. Knowing that cancer is still present, the doctor has several methods and treatments to control it as much as possible.

Angiogenesis

When you think about it, setting up a distant colony is a remarkable feat. This cell, or a few cells, float around in the blood stream, then find a suitable spot and settle down. A few cells can exist for a while by diffusion of nutrition from existing blood vessels. But as they multiply and grow they need an ever increasing and constant supply of blood to bring oxygen and food for their voracious appetites. But the lack of blood vessels is not much of a problem for the pioneer cells. They simply secrete substances that the nearest blood vessels pick up. These substances, Vascular Epithelial Growth Factors (VEGF), cause the nearby blood vessels to create a new path to the metastatic colony. This is called angiogenesis. (*Angio* is from the Greek, meaning vessel,—*genesis* is from the Greek meaning generation or birth).

Over 40 angiogenesis-inducing compounds have been identified. Several anti-angiogenesis compounds have been discovered. These substances seem to work well in stopping cancer growth in animals. Lots of promising research is being done.

Oncologist

An oncologist is a doctor who specializes in the management or treatment of cancer. *Onkos* is from the Greek, which means tumor or mass.

Adenocarcinoma

Adeno—means gland. Since the prostate is a gland, prostate cancers are called prostatic adenocarcinomas. An adenocarcinoma could occur in any gland, such as the adrenals, the thyroid or the pancreas. A gland is usually an organ or structure that produces and secretes substances that may be used in other parts of the body.

Chromosomes

Your body is made up of several trillion very tiny cells. The cells have a central nucleus which contains the chromosomes, protoplasm and other structures. The chromosomes carry the 40,000 genes that determine the characteristics of the person. There are various numbers of chromosomes in the cells of different plants and animals. In the human, there are 23 pairs. These pairs of chromosomes are called diploid, which simply means twofold. Diploidy means that the cells have two sets of homologous chromosomes. Homologous means that they are similar, such as your two hands are similar.

Some cancer cells do not have the characteristic pairs of chromosomes. Some of them may be aneuploid, (the prefix *an*—means without or not, *eu* means good), which means that the cells are not good and do not have the normal pairs of chromosomes. A single cancerous tumor may have several different ploidy types of cells. Ploidy tests can be done on biopsied material from a tumor to determine the ploidy. Those tumors that have a high percentage of aneuploidy usually have a poor prognosis. (*Prognosis* is from the Greek meaning foreknowledge. It usually means a prediction of an outcome of a disease).

CANCER PREVENTION

We still don't know all of the factors involved in the causes of cancer. Of course you need to avoid the known carcinogens. Until we fully understand the causes of cancer, it is difficult to prevent it. That is especially so for prostate cancer.

A dietary study of 47,000 men over a six year period, done at Harvard, was published in the Dec. 1995 Journal of the National Institute. It showed that men who eat at least ten servings a week of tomatoes or tomato based foods such as pizza and spaghetti sauce were 45% less likely to develop prostate cancer. It is the lycopenes in the tomatoes. Several other vegetables also contain lycopenes.

Some studies have linked high animal fats to breast and prostate cancer. There are several different types of fats. Dr. Charles Myers, who wrote part of Chapter 19 on Diet and Exercise, has done a lot of study on the various types of fats. Check out what he has to say about the various types of fats.

Low levels of minerals such as zinc and selenium have been cited as a possible cause of prostate cancer. Dr. L. C. Clark did a comprehensive study on selenium. His study indicated that 200 ug of selenium per day could help prevent prostate cancer. Selenium supplementation may reduce the risk of certain cancers, according to a study published in the Dec. 25, 1997, issue of the Journal of the American Medical Association (JAMA). The study included data on 1,312 patients over a 10-year period. While there was no decrease in skin cancers, there was a 40 percent decrease in overall cancer risk, with marked decreases in the incidence of lung, colorectal and prostate cancer. To find out more about selenium studies, go to www.yahoo.com, www.google.com or any of the other search engines, and search for selenium AND prostate cancer. You can use the search engines to find data about almost anything you would like.

Testosterone levels may also be suspect in the cause of prostate cancer. Oriental men usually have a fairly low level of testosterone compared to Caucasians. Black men usually have a rather high level. We know that prostate cancer is dependent on testosterone. If a male is castrated early in life, he will never have prostate cancer or benign prostatic hyperplasia (BPH).

One of the most effective treatments for prostate cancer that has metastasized is castration. (A more euphemistic term is orchiectomy, but it means the same thing.) A less harsh treatment is to use drugs that chemically counteract androgenic hormone productions and bring them down to castrate level. These drugs are usually very expensive compared to orchiectomy. But most men would rather hold onto their family jewels because they represent manhood. Even if the testicles are nothing but a useless ornament that no one will ever see, they still want to keep them. Besides, maybe they will get lucky and their cancer will go into remission. Or someone will come up with a magic bullet, a miracle cure.

There is a lot of variation in testosterone levels, by age and throughout the day. The highest levels are usually in the morning. On average, testosterone levels change with age. The highest level is from about 15 years old up to 30 years old, then it starts drop-ping. The levels may range from 400 ng/100 ml (nanograms per milliliter) up to 1100 ng/100 ml at age 30. At age 70 it may range from 200 ng/100 ml up to about 600 ng/100 ml. For men who are undergoing combined hormone therapy (CHT), the goal is to bring the testosterone level down to 20ng/100ml or less. This is consid-ered to be castrate level.

Prostate cancer is related to testosterone, but it seems strange that more men get the cancer when they are older and the test-osterone levels are normally decreasing. In a similar manner, more women get breast cancer after they have experienced menopause and are no longer producing estrogen. One possible reason could be that the beginning prostate cancer and breast cancer may have started several years earlier when the person was producing large amounts of the hormones.

Several genetic studies are being done to find new methods of early detection of certain cancers. The researchers can look at the genes and detect differences that may predispose the person to cancer long before it becomes evident. But several questions have been raised. What happens if a person is told that they have a high risk of developing cancer and he or she tries to buy health insur-ance? What happens to their employment? What will be the rules of privacy? What happens to his state of mind if he is told that he will die an early death because of cancer?

Dr. David Bostwick, and others, have found that High Grade Pros-tate Intraepithelial Neoplasia (HGPIN) may be a precursor to pros-tate cancer that can be detected by a biopsy. The biopsy may not detect any cancer, but some of the cells may show that they are changing and undergoing HGPIN. Dr. Bostwick has treated some of his patients who had HGPIN with Proscar and Casodex and they do not progress to prostate cancer. There have not been a lot of stud-ies done yet, but it would seem to be a way to prevent prostate cancer.

HOW WE START LIFE

We first start life as a single cell that results from the uniting of a single sperm from the father and an egg from the mother. Neither the sperm nor the egg is a complete cell by itself. Every cell in our body has 46 chromosomes except that the sperm and egg cells have 23 chromosomes each. When the sperm and egg unite they form a complete cell which will have 46 chromosomes. (Different animals and plants may have a different number of chromosomes.)

The chromosomes contain the genetic material, inherited from each of your parents, that determines who you are and what you are.

Once the sperm and egg have united, almost immediately the single cell begins to divide and multiply. It divides into two complete cells, these two become four, the four become eight. Soon the single cell that resulted from the union of the sperm and egg becomes an embryo that has millions of cells.

To give you an idea of how cells multiply here is an old problem. It asked, "Which would you choose, to be given one million dollars outright, or to be given a single penny, then have it doubled each day for 30 days?" Without doing the simple math, many people would say they would rather have the million dollars. But if you are given one penny on the first day, then two on the second day, four on the third, and continue to double the amount each day, on the 30th day the single penny doubled each day would amount to $5,368,709.12. On the 31st day the amount would be $10,737,418.24.

The cells in the embryo may double and multiply even more often than once a day, so it is easy to understand how one cell can quickly develop into trillions. But the fast-growing cells in the developing embryo are strictly regulated and controlled. After the baby is born, the cells continue to rapidly grow and multiply until the person reaches adulthood when normal growth is stopped and cells will only be produced to repair or replace damaged or worn out tissues. At this time the body will be made up of the several trillion cells.

DIFFERENTIATION

The body is made up of several different cells, organs and tissues. All of these different cells are derived from the single cell that resulted from the fertilized egg. As the embryo grows and develops, the cells change, or **differentiate**, into whatever cell type is needed for a particular tissue or organ.

It is interesting to note that some plants and lower animals retain a large amount of undifferentiated cells throughout life. There are so many undifferentiated cells in some plants, such as the geranium, that all you need is a small piece of a branch to grow or clone a complete new plant. Some lizards can lose a part of their tail or a foot to a predator and the tail or foot will eventually regrow from embryonic type undifferentiated cells. If we could find out how the lower animals do this, perhaps humans could do it. Studies are being done using human embryonic tissues, even though some people are protesting such studies.

When a cancer develops, the cells may have several different shapes and forms. Some of the cancer cells may be very similar to the original prostate or whatever type of tissue it derived from. These cells would be called well differentiated. Some of the cells within the tumor may not have any resemblance at all to the original cells. These would be called poorly differentiated or undifferentiated. Between these two extremes might be some moderately differentiated cells. The process of cells becoming poorly differentiated or undifferentiated is sometimes called dedifferentiation.

Most prostate cancers may have a mix of many different stages of differentiation. The Gleason Score for staging prostate cancer is based on the mix of the differentiation of the cells. We will discuss the Gleason Score in Chapter Six.

Ordinarily, those tumors with a large number of poorly differentiated cells are the more aggressive and dangerous. They grow faster and metastasize early. They usually have a worse prognosis than the well differentiated type tumors. But this is not always the case. There are no hard and fast rules that are etched in stone when it comes to cancer. Again, the only rule regarding cancer is that there are no rules. There are exceptions and sometimes the poorly differentiated tumor may grow no faster than a tumor that is well differentiated. And sometimes the well differentiated may become aggressive and fast growing.

FOUR BASIC FUNCTIONS OF LIFE

Together, our many cells form a complete system or person. There are four basic functions that we all do. We eat, we digest the food, we eliminate the waste and we reproduce. Each of the individual cells in your body performs the same basic functions. Food and oxygen is brought to each cell by the blood stream. The cell takes in the nutrition, digests it, then throws off the waste products into the lymph system, the clear fluid that surrounds each cell.

Each individual cell has a purpose and a job to do. Depending on what part of the system they are, every one of our cells perform specific functions that keep us alive. For instance, the cells in the lungs take the oxygen that we breathe in and throws off the carbon dioxide waste. The cells of the stomach and intestines produce enzymes and chemicals to help break down and digest the food we eat so that it can be used by the various other cells of the body. Cells in glands such as the pituitary, the adrenals, the ovaries and testes produce hormones that are vital to us in controlling our bodies.

Even the lowly cells that make up our skin have several purposes and functions. Among the many jobs the skin does is to cover and protect our vital organs. It helps to protect us from the invasion of infectious organisms. It also acts a barrier to many chemicals and toxic materials. It contains many of the sensory nerve fibers that allow us to feel and to be aware of our environment. It helps maintain body temperature by perspiration and has many other functions.

THE BLOOD AND LYMPH SYSTEM

In order for any cell or tissue to survive and grow it must have a constant supply of food and oxygen. There must also be a means to remove the waste products. The blood and lymph system perform these tasks.

The heart circulates the blood through the lungs where it throws off waste carbon dioxide and picks up oxygen. It pumps the freshly oxygenated blood out to all of the tissues and cells of the body, drops off the oxygen and picks up the waste carbon dioxide. Some of the blood is also circulated around the intestines to pick up nutrition and deliver it to the cells that need it. The blood-stream also picks up hormones and enzymes and delivers them to the tissues where they are needed.

When the blood leaves the heart, it is under a considerable amount of pressure. The arteries leaving the heart are fairly large. But as they branch down into the very small capillaries there is very little pressure left when they connect to the venous blood vessels. The venous blood vessels rely primarily on a one-way valve system to get the blood back to the heart. Most veins have muscles near them or that surround them. When a muscle is contracted it squeezes on the vein and forces the blood toward the heart.

When the muscle is relaxed, the blood may try to fall back, but a small flap or valve in the vein closes and prevents the blood from going backwards.

The lymph system is a system of vessels very much like the venous system. The vessels have one-way valves much like the veins. A major difference in the veins and the lymph system is that the blood system is a closed system, the veins connect directly to the arteries through the capillaries. The lymph system is open on the collecting end. The cells dump the waste, or end products of digestion and metabolism, into the surrounding lymph fluid.

Much like the venous system, when a muscle is flexed, the lymph fluid is forced through the one-way valves of the lymph vessels.

This waste material is dumped into the venous system near the heart.

LYMPH NODES

One of the tests to determine whether a cancer has metastasized is to examine the nearby lymph nodes. The lymph system is somewhat similar to the drainage system of our streets. When it rains, water flows into drainage pipes below the streets. Steel grates filter out the large waste materials. In our lymph system, a series of nodes filter out bacteria and any foreign agents to prevent them from getting into the blood stream. The lymph nodes produce special cells that can kill off bacteria and help maintain the body's immune system. Quite often the lymph nodes will become enlarged whenever a person becomes ill. The nodes will produce large numbers of killer cells to try to protect the body.

HOW CANCER SPREADS

Whenever cancer starts to spread, some of the metastatic cells are often stopped temporarily by lymph nodes. But the cancer cells usually don't cause enough alarm to cause the lymph nodes to stop them completely. The lymph nodes may become overwhelmed and the cancer cells may proceed on their way to set up new colonies or tumors. In prostate cancer, quite often the new metastatic tumors are formed in the bones of the spine.

When a radical prostatectomy is performed, ordinarily, the lymph nodes are examined first for cancerous cells. A microscopic examination of the lymph nodes can often reveal whether a cancer has metastasized. Sometimes a laparoscopic examination will be done before the operation. Or the surgeon will take out the lymph nodes and have a pathologist examine them immediately.

If any cancer cells are found in the lymph nodes, it means that the cancer has already spread. In this case, it usually doesn't help to remove the prostate. Like the old saying, it's not much use locking the barn door after the horse has escaped. Most doctors will sew the patient back up and start him on other therapy. However, a recent study reveals that removing the prostate and starting the patient immediately on hormone therapy improves survival when compared to removing the prostate and delaying hormone therapy.

The cancer cells may also escape through the many blood vessels that enter and leave the prostate. A prostate cancer cell may be no bigger than a blood cell, so it would be no problem to travel along with them.

There are also lots of nerves that enter and leave the prostate. Quite often perineural invasion is found in removed prostates. Which means that the cancer cells were found migrating in the sheath that surrounds nerves. (Perineural—*peri* means around, *neural* means nerve.)

The other way for the cells to escape is through extension and invasion. Remember that cancer means crab. The cancer may send out fingers of cells that penetrate the prostatic capsule and enter the nearby pelvic organs such as the seminal vesicles.

As long as the cancer is contained, stays fairly small, and does not invade a vital organ, it may not kill the host. The cancer usually kills when it gets so large that it is an unbearable burden to the body. It can also kill when it invades an organ that is vital to life such as the lungs or brain. Often when it invades another organ, it usually grows to such an extent that it crowds out all of the normal cells. The cancer cells have a voracious appetite and may deprive the normal cells of any available nutrition.

Cancer may also kill by debilitation of the patient. They may not even be able to determine the source of the cancer, but the patient may become weak, lose weight and gradually fade away.

HOW CANCER SURVIVES

At the present time when cancer is diagnosed, we have no way of knowing whether it has already set up micrometastases somewhere in the body. We do know that if the PSA is 20 or greater and the Gleason score is more than 7, the cancer has probably already escaped the prostate gland.

Because we can't recognize early metastatic disease, some men are operated on needlessly. Some of these men may appear to have been cured, but within five years, metastatic cancer may become evident in up to 20 percent or more of men who were thought to have been cured. The final pathology report on the removed prostate and Gleason sum can sometimes predict who will fail.

Reverse transcriptase polymerase chain reaction (RTPCR) is a test that can detect cancer cells in the blood-stream. But just being able to find a cancer cell in the blood-stream is no guarantee that it will be able to find a suitable place to settle down, establish a colony and grow new blood vessels.

When cancer cells begin to proliferate, they must have lots of food and nutrition. To get it requires extra blood and lymph vessels. The ingenious cancer cells produce angiogenic factors that cause the body to create the extra blood and lymph vessels.

For every chemical, drug or hormone that causes an action, there is usually one that causes an opposite reaction. Scientists have discovered several of the tumor angiogenic factors. Several studies are being done with anti-angiogenic drugs that would inhibit the production of the angiogenic factors. By counteracting the angiogenic factors produced by the cancer cells, they would be denied a blood supply and nutrition and would thus die.

ONCOGENES

There are about 40,000 genes in the 46 chromosomes of each cell. The genes are carried in the DNA and are the blueprint of all the characteristics that were inherited from the parents. The genes determine the eye color, the person's size and shape and all of the characteristics of a person. Some studies have indicated that a few of these genes, about 100 or so, are oncogenes, or genes that can cause cancer.

The cells of our body normally reproduce or split exactly in half when it is necessary to replace or repair nearby cells or tissues. When oncogenes are "hit" by a carcinogen, then reproduce, the resulting new cells may be abnormal cancer cells. Some studies seem to indicate that it may take two or more hits to the oncogenes from carcinogens to cause cancer.

CANCER AND AGE

Another factor in cancer is the person's age. The older a person is, the more likely that the person's oncogenes have endured several "hits" in his or her lifetime. So it is more likely that the older person will develop cancer. This is especially so for most breast and prostate cancer victims who are usually over 50 years old.

But many younger people also get cancer. Quite often, when cancer develops in a younger person, it is usually very aggressive and more likely to metastasize. It may be that the younger person sustained a direct hit from a strong carcinogen to their oncogenes. Another reason may be that the person, young or old, may have inherited certain genetic flaws that predispose the person to have cancer.

There are thousands of carcinogenic factors. We are besieged by them on every side, in our homes, the workplace, in the air we breathe, in our food and in the genes we inherited from our parents and ancestors. We may never be able to identify all of the carcinogens. Even if we could identify all of them, there is no way we could protect ourselves from them and still live a normal life.

DNA REPAIR

The body is a very adaptable machine. The older person's system may learn to adapt and live with several small doses of carcinogens. The DNA of a normal cell can repair the genetic damage if it is not too severe. It is when the body is overwhelmed that our defense systems break down and the body is overcome. One reason that radiation treatments kill cancer cells is that the cancer cells do not have the ability to repair the damage done to them.

PROGRAMMED CELL DEATH, APOPTOSIS

Remember that all of the many trillions of cells in your body are derived from the original egg and sperm cell. Remember that the cells in your body must constantly replace any damaged cells, the old worn out cells, and cells needed for growth. Some studies have indicated that there is a finite number of times the cells can reproduce. It appears that the cells are programmed to die when this limit is reached. Scientists have called it apoptosis. The upper age limit for man seems to be about 120 years. Inherited genes are a big factor. So is the environment the body is subjected to and many other factors.

When a cell dies due to injury or some toxic substance, there is often an alarm.

It causes swelling, redness and other effects of the damage. This alerts the bodies defenses and macrophages and other large cells rapidly move in and clean up the dead cells. Apoptosis, or natural death, does not cause any alarm but it does cause the macrophages and other cells to clean up and remove the waste products.

As we get older, the cells that have changed and adapted make us into a different person. Because we are in a constant state of change and flux, we are a different person each day of our lives.

HOW CANCER MAY START

Our bodies are made up of several hundred trillion separate individual living cells. (A trillion is 1,000,000,000,000). Most of the cells are so small that thousands of them could fit in the space occupied by the period at the end of this sentence. Examples of cells are the skin cells, muscle cells, nerve cells and other cells that make up the different tissues and organs of the body.

The various cells form tissues, glands, organs and systems. Each cell, gland and organ has a purpose and a function. They all work together to form a complete system that sustains us and keeps us alive. All of these different cells are derived from the first complete cell that was formed from the sperm and the ovum. The sperm and the ovum each contributed 23 chromosomes to make the complete cell with 46 chromosomes. Each of the cells in our bodies, whether prostate, liver or lung each have copies of the original 46 chromosomes.

Occasionally some of the cells wear out, are damaged, or for some reason die off. Even the cells in a young baby may wear out or become damaged. Sometimes a large number of cells are killed off or attacked by an infectious or harmful agent. Our bodies are marvelous machines and we have several defenses. Unless the damage or the attack is overwhelming, we can usually overcome the injury and recover our health.

In most instances, the cells that are killed off or damaged are replaced by nearby cells. A nearby cell of the same type as those damaged or killed off, will simply split in half and become two cells. The normal cells will continue to divide and multiply until the damage is repaired and then stop reproducing.

Occasionally something may happen to cause one of these reproducing cells not to divide exactly in half. A daughter cell may not get exactly half of the chromosomes. Or the chromosomes may be damaged in some way. The resulting cells are no longer like any of the normal cells in our body. Often, the body will recognize these aberrant cells and destroy them. Unfortunately, some of them may not be recognized, and they begin dividing and creating more and more of the abnormal cells. The body stops the reproduction of the normal cell when they are no longer needed. But it has no control at all over the abnormal cancer cell growth.

The cancer cells do not perform any useful function. They contribute nothing to the system. They take more than their share of nutrition, often robbing the neighboring hard-working cells of their nutrition. They are parasites that often grow so large that they squeeze the neighboring tissues and kill them off.

Normal cells have a definite life span with programmed death or apoptosis. From laboratory studies, it appears that normal cells can divide about 50 times before they die. But instead of living for a certain length of time, then dying off, cancer cells keep right on living and multiplying into new cells that refuse to die. They are, in effect, immortal.

One reason may be because of telomeres. There is a section called a telomere (*telos* is Greek for end, *meros* is part) at the end of the chromosomes. It appears from some studies that the telomere becomes a bit shorter each time a cell divides. When the telomere decreases to a certain length, the cell dies from the programmed death called apoptosis.

Scientists have discovered that most all cancer cells cause an enzyme, telomerase, to be produced. Telomerase prevents the telomere from being shortened or affected when the cell divides. This appears to be what makes the cancer cell immortal.

Scientists have found telomerase present in 90% of all cancers. They hope that the presence of telomerase can be used as a marker for early detection of cancers. It might also be used to determine the aggressiveness of cancers. Scientists are searching for a substance that can counteract the telomerase enzyme. Without the telomerase, the cancer cells would eventually die off just like normal cells.

CANCER GROWTH

The transformation of a single cell into one million cells would be too small to be detectable by most methods. Remember the doubling of the penny, over one million cells would be created after only 20 doublings. After 30 doublings, the tumor would have over one billion cells and could be detected as a lump. After it had doubled 40 times, the tumor would have about 1,099,511,627,780 or one trillion, 99 billion, 511 million, 627 thousand and 780 cells. The tumor would weigh about two pounds.

Depending on the type of cancer, its location and how aggressive it is, it may take years for it to double 20 or 30 times and reach a size to where it can be detected. During this time, it may not cause any pain or alarm to the body. A tumor may only cause pain or dysfunction if it is located in or near a vital organ. In this case its presence may be detected before it has doubled more than 30 times.

OVER 100 DIFFERENT FORMS OF CANCER

One reason it is difficult to find cancer before it has spread is that cancer is not a single disease. Cancer can arise in any of the cells, tissues, glands or organs of the body. Over 100 different forms of cancer have been identified.

There is some indication that there may be at least three different and distinct types of prostate cancer. The most prevalent type is a latent form which may never cause any problems. These cancers have a very low PSA and a low Gleason score. The moderate type may have a Gleason score of 5 to 7 and a PSA up to 10. It can progress and may eventually kill one. The very aggressive type may have a PSA of 20 or so and a Gleason score of 8 to 10. Its PSA may have a short doubling time and it may kill within just a few years.

ORIGIN AND GROWTH

Cancers usually arise at a primary site such as the prostate gland, the lungs, stomach or intestines. Cancer may remain at its original site and simply grow into a small tumor. You may have it for years and never know it. Eventually it may become a large tumor.

A cancer patient needs to make sure that his or her body gets plenty of the proper nutrition every day. The patient must intake enough nutrition, not only to satisfy the greedy and voracious appetite of the cancer cells, but to also have enough left over to feed and repair the normal cells.

Unfortunately, in many cases of advanced cancer, the person may lose his or her appetite completely. It is believed that the appetite loss is due to some factor produced by the cancer cells. The patient loses weight and may be just skin and bones when the cancer finally overwhelms and kills him or her.

A DETAILED EXPLANATION OF METASTASES

Dr. Roger Sopher is with the University of North Dakota School of Medicine, Department of Pathology. He is a prostate cancer survivor and devotes a lot of time answering questions on the Internet.

> <<Meir Pann said: My point is, in all these years, wouldn't an errant cell or two be released, to wander in this universe of me, and be established somewhere as a micro-metastasis? Couldn't we point to this possibility as a source of the large percentage of the failed RPs on "localized, contained tumor" we see years after the operation?>>

Here is Dr. Sopher's reply:

> "You have it pretty close to right but as you might guess it is an incredibly complex set of interconnecting events. The basic idea is that a single cell develops the capability of malignant behavior through a series of mutations. Some of these mutations were passed down from precursor cells that had only a partial change in their genome and some occurred in the final stage of things.

> One of the things that happens in cells that have become malignant is that they lose the normal mechanisms that screen the genome for mistakes. Without these screening mechanisms, additional mutations become even easier and more prevalent. The term used is that cancer cells are genetically labile which means that they are easily changeable. As the clones of malignant cells develop, subclones also are produced. Many of these have lethal mutations and they die. But some have mutations that give the malignant cells some selective advantage in growth. Generally when this happens the subclones are worse behaved than their progenitors. This is termed tumor progression.

> Now, a malignant tumor can only achieve a size of a couple of millimeters without its own blood supply. This was shown by a surgeon, Judah Folkman, in the seventies.(Editor's Note: In 1998, Dr. Folkman proved that he could cure cancer in mice by using endostatin and angiostatin. Several human trials are ongoing at the present time. We are confident that it will cure some cancers in humans). The tumor is incapable of making

blood vessels. But it does have the ability to co-opt the surrounding stroma (connective tissue) into producing blood vessels for it by releasing a number of chemical signals.

At the same time the tumor often causes a particular kind of inflammatory cell (the macrophage) to come into the area. Macrophages, when they are activated, also produce chemical signals that cause the formation of blood vessels. The net effect is that the cells that should be involved in killing tumor cells help produce what the tumor needs to grow—blood vessels.

Now that the tumor has its blood supply, it can achieve greater and continued growth. Additional subclones develop that have the ability to invade through the walls of blood vessels. Clumps of tumor cells then can break off and circulate. As they float along they are generally covered by a layer of plasma proteins and platelets that hides them from the immune system.

The tumor cells have receptors on their surface that can bind to specific sites on the endothelial surface (lining of the blood vessels) that allows them to grab on.

In some cases the physical size of the tumor clumps stops their progression through the microvasculature on the basis of size and they form a plug.

Some tumors definitely have the ability to home to specific sites for reasons that are still not completely understood. For example prostate cancer cells like to go to bone as does breast cancer cells. Lung tumors like bone, the adrenal glands, the brain and many other sites.

We know that tumors shed cells into the circulation even before any metastatic sites can be demonstrated. This was shown nicely in the mid 80s in breast cancer. Some women had no involvement in their regional lymph nodes. When their bone marrow was sampled at the time of surgery and then analyzed, between 15 and 20 percent of these women had cancer cells in their bone marrow. In a follow up, there was no good correlation between the women that had cancer cells in their marrow at the time of surgery and those that went on to develop progressive disease.

So the mere fact that tumor cells are in the circulation does not seem to be a good predictor of those that will develop metastatic disease. The reverse transcriptase polymerase chain reaction (RTPCR) test has been used to probe for circulating prostate cells in the blood stream. It is a very sensitive test. In theory one can pick up a single cell in a 10 ml sample of blood. The problem is, what does it mean? At this point, in my view, not much until some correlation with progressive disease can be proved. UCLA has recently done a study of RTPCR and came to the same conclusion.

Some believe that a primary tumor may produce an angiostatin substance which may help keep other tumors in check. Angiostatin certainly exists and may explain the rare case in which metastatic sites "blossom" when the main tumor is removed or conversely regresses. However those events are not common.

One of the interesting things about tumor growth is that it is not a linear function. Work done at the Argonne National Laboratory has suggested that tumor growth follows a Gompertz curve which says that it starts off fast and then slows down fast. The slowing is thought to be on the basis of the intrinsically poor blood supply of most tumors. When a metastasis occurs, it tends to grow as a new colony and follows its own Gompertz curve. Therapies aimed at preventing the tumor from inducing angiogenesis are very exciting. They may not cure anyone of the tumor but they would, in theory, make its presence inconsequential.

Our knowledge of basic tumor biology is improving. With the advances in molecular biology we are starting to understand things that were not even dreamed of just a few years ago. As a cancer patient, it may not seem like it, but we are gaining in our war. However, we still have many battles to wage."

Roger L. Sopher, MD

Dept of Pathology

University of North Dakota School of Medicine, Grand Forks, ND

58202-9037

TREATMENT CHOICES

If a person is told that he has cancer, even if it is a small slow growing one, it may cause a lot of worry and stress. He may insist on having it treated or removed. If the operation is done properly and early enough, the person may live longer than a person who has never had cancer. The reason for a longer life is that the person may start taking better care of himself.

If the cancer is fairly small, at T1a or T2b stage and the biopsy shows a low Gleason grade, the doctor may recommend that the tumor just be closely watched and monitored. If there is any change in the PSA or the other prostate tests, then treatment can be instituted immediately. If the person is over 75 years old, and the cancer seems to be growing slowly, the doctor may also recommend that it just be watched and closely monitored.

If it appears that the patient has less than ten years to live, most doctors will not recommend a prostatectomy. Instead if the patient is elderly or in poor health he may be given Hormone Therapy. He may also be offered other forms of treatment that are not quite as traumatic as radical surgery such as Cryosurgery, Brachytherapy or Seed Implants, External Beam Radiation (XBRT), or Proton Beam irradiation. For advanced disease, the patient may be offered various forms of chemotherapy.

You should always remember though, no matter what the doctor recommends, it is your body, your disease and your choice of treatments. Of course, you should take into consideration that the doctor should know more than you do. But if you ask ten doctors what the best treatment would be, you may get ten different answers. You must endeavor to learn all you can, then make your own decision.

In Greek mythology, Aphrodite, the goddess of beauty and love, sprang fully grown and mature at birth. Unlike Aphrodite, cancer starts from a single cell and grows. Your cancer is not going to kill you overnight. It may have taken 10 years or more to become significant enough to be detected. You have a bit of time to do your study. Don't let anyone rush you into a treatment that you may regret later. A very important part of your decision is choosing the best doctor.

CANCER IS NOT CONTAGIOUS

Cancer may cause some people to avoid or shun a cancer victim or to be afraid of them. But cancer is not contagious. It cannot be transmitted to another person. Cancer is nothing more than a few of the body's own cells that have begun to multiply abnormally. Cancer can only derive from the cells in your body.

CANCER AND PAIN

Some cancers can be terribly painful, disabling and traumatic, not only to the person who has it, but to the whole family. If a close friend or relative is suffering, you may also suffer right along with them.

If the cancer is causing a lot of pain, there are several things that a doctor can do to alleviate the pain. Sometimes radiation will help. Sometimes it may be necessary to use morphine and other strong pain killers. Often metastatic prostate cancer spreads to the bones and causes great pain. A radioactive isotope strontium 89 can often relieve the pain. Some chemotherapy drugs are good at relieving pain caused by metastases.

There are some cancers that cause no pain or alarm at all until they have spread and metastasized. Since they cause no pain or alarm to the body, it is often difficult to find them before it is too late to properly treat them. Many cancers are not life threatening. For instance, if the cancer remains contained in the prostate, it may never cause any problems.

SOME CANCER SIGNS

Here are some signs that should cause suspicion of cancer in men, women or children: Any increased skin pigmentation, a sore that does not heal, unusual bleeding, a thickening or a lump in the breast or anywhere in the body, indigestion or difficulty in swallowing, rectal bleeding, a change in the bowel habits that persists, shortness of breath, fatigue, change in a wart or mole, bone pain, frequent urination, and decreased urinary stream.

Having one or more of these symptoms does not necessarily mean that you have cancer. Or you may have none of the above symptoms and still have cancer. It can be a silent killer. But it is very easy to get checked out. We will say it again and again. If the cancer is found early enough, it can usually be cured. The answer to cancer is early detection.

CANCER AND YOU

It appears that some prostate cancers may be caused by some environmental factors and perhaps diet. A recent study done by Dr. Edward Giovannucci at Harvard Medical School seems to indicate that fats from red meats are a contributing factor in prostate cancer. Animal fats are also highly suspect as a factor in breast cancer development.

In Japan clinical stage prostate cancer is very low. But if Japanese come to the United States, their rate is about the same as for Caucasians. When autopsies are done on Japanese men in Japan they find about the same rate of undetected prostate cancer as that of American men. Because of the crowded conditions in Japan, they have very little land on which to grow cattle. Most meat is imported and is very expensive. So most families eat very little meat. Instead they eat a lot of fish and soy products.

We do know that there is one thing that does not cause prostate cancer. That is sex. Even overindulgence in sex acts of any kind or masturbation does not cause prostate cancer. This is one area where you can't get too much of a good thing.

CAUSES OF DEATH

Ordinarily, cancer cells alone do not cause death. The body is a fantastic machine. It is also very adaptable and can survive and overcome unbelievable traumas and injuries.

Unless the cancer destroys a vital organ such as the brain, lungs or heart, it does not directly kill the host. It may kill by cachexia (*kakos* is Greek for bad, *hexis* means condition). Cachexia is a state of ill health, malnutrition and wasting. Many cancer patients lose their appetite which causes malnutrition. It appears that the tumors may produce factors that cause cachexia.

When prostate and breast cancers metastasize, the cells often set up new colonies in the bones of the vertebrae. The bones may become eroded. The calcium from the eroded bones may be taken up by the blood stream. The body must have a certain amount of calcium. But if there is too much in the blood stream, it may cause hypercalcemia.

Hypercalcemia may cause a change in mental alertness, anorexia, nausea, vomiting, constipation, excessive thirst, frequent urination, muscle weakness and a diminished muscle reflex. Kidney failure is common. Hypercalcemia is very serious and is associated with a high mortality rate. Prostate cancer may also cause blood coagulation problems and anemia.

In an old classic textbook, a fifth edition of *Boyd's Textbook of Pathology*, published in 1947 by Lea & Febiger, Philadelphia. The following is quoted from this book, page 14:

> "...disease is not a state; it is rather a process ever changing in its manifestations, a process which may end in recovery or in death, which may be acute and fulminating in its manifestations, or which may represent the slow ageing of the tissues brought about by the sharp tooth of time....(a) lesion (may have) been present during many years of life, and its presence is not sufficient to explain the final end....the pathologist has to try to explain not only why the patient died but how he was able to live." As Boycott remarks (Lancet, 1933, 2, 846) "I do not wonder that people die; that is easy enough. What I marvel at is that they go on living with bodies so maimed, so disordered and worn out."

One factor that makes prostate cancer so life threatening is that it affects mostly older men. The "sharp tooth" of time has dulled and weakened their normal body defenses. Thus they may be more susceptible, and less immune, to the many lesser infections and opportunistic diseases.

Chapter Three

MY PROSTATE CANCER

Dr. Aubrey Pilgrim

I was almost 68 years old. I had been having trouble urinating for some time. I had a very small stream. Even after I had urinated I often felt like I still needed to go. I had to get up frequently at night to urinate.

After I urinated, I could stand there and shake it for five minutes. But the second that I put it back in my pants, it would dribble all over me. It was quite embarrassing.

I also noticed that I was having more trouble having sex. My wife died in 1986 after over 42 years of marriage. I have not re-married, but I love sex, so I had a lady friend.

DIGITAL RECTAL EXAM (DRE) & PSA TEST

I finally went to see my doctor, an HMO internist. He did a digital rectal exam (DRE) and said that my prostate seemed a bit enlarged, but he didn't seem to be too concerned. I had heard about the prostate specific antigen (PSA) test and asked him if I should have one. He said that test was for suspected cases of prostate cancer and didn't seem to think that I needed it.

I insisted on having a PSA test so he referred me to a urologist. The urologist did another DRE on me and said that my prostate was about four times larger than it should be. He seemed to be concerned and sent me to the blood lab for a PSA test.

URINE RETENTION TEST

The urologist also sent me to have a urine retention test. This test checks to see if all of the urine is voided from the bladder each time you go. The prostate has a tough capsule that surrounds it. The prostate may grow so large that it can squeeze and close off the urinary canal that passes through it. One may not be able to completely empty the bladder and urine may be retained in the bladder. Depending on the amount of retention, it can cause kidney problems, bladder infections and other problems.

To check for urine retention, I was given a drink that had a dye in it. The dye can be seen with X-rays. After a period of time, I was asked to void, then an X-ray was taken of my bladder. It proved that I was retaining a large amount of urine. This is known as residual urine.

BPH

The doctor said not to worry, that it may be only benign prostatic hyperplasia (BPH) growth. (It is sometimes called hypertrophy instead of hyperplasia. Hyperplasia is the better term since it means excessive growth or proliferation of normal tissue cells. Hypertrophy means excessive nourishment.)

It was easy enough for him to say, "Don't worry". BPH occurs in most older men. The BPH growth is made up of non-cancerous cells. It is a fairly simple operation to perform a "Roto Rooter" procedure to ream out and open up the urinary duct. The proper term for the procedure is Transurethral Resection of the Prostate or TURP. The device is inserted into the urethra of the penis and some of the obstructing tissue is trimmed away. They can also use laser and other procedures to trim away prostatic tissue and open the urethra. I was hoping very much that my problem was only a BPH growth. (We will discuss BPH in depth in Chapter Five.)

I went back a week later for the PSA results. It was 10.2 ng/ml. The normal figure for my age would be less than 4 ng/ml. I don't have to tell you that I was a bit worried. My urologist was not very communicative. He set up an appointment for a biopsy. I asked a few questions, but I just couldn't force myself to say the word "cancer." So I went home and worried. And worried.

BIOPSY

I went back a week later for the biopsy. It is a relatively painless procedure. A device with a spring-loaded needle is inserted into the rectum. The needle pierces the rectal wall and into the prostate gland. The needle picks up a few cells. He took two samples of tissue, one from each rear lobe of the prostate. The samples were sent to a laboratory for analysis by a pathologist.

The needle can miss some cancers, especially a smaller tumor. Some doctors may take six or more samples just to make sure. Some prostate cancers may be made up of as many as six or more small colonies.

My doctor was not up on the latest technologies and procedures in a lot of ways. The large bore spring loaded needle that he used was practically obsolete. Many of the newer systems use a much smaller needle. Most doctors also use Transrectal Ultrasound (TRUS) to view the prostate and to guide the needle. Many small tumors that can't be felt can be visualized with ultra sound. My prostate cancer lumps could be easily felt so that the doctor hit paydirt on both sticks.

BLEEDING DURING SEX

The doctor told me that after the biopsy I might have blood in my urine for a while so I wasn't too surprised when I saw the blood. I didn't see any more blood in my urine after about a week so I persuaded my lady friend to have sex. I was anxious to have as much sex as possible because I was afraid that it might be my last time.

After we had sex, my lady friend went to the bathroom. There was blood all over her. She panicked. I didn't feel too good about the situation either. But she was very concerned that the blood might have cancer cells in it, which might somehow infect her. Such a thing is absolutely impossible.

THE BIOPSY RESULTS, CANCER

It took about two weeks to get the biopsy test results. I worried myself sick while waiting. I finally got a call to come see the doctor. When he came into the room he didn't have to tell me. I could see it in his face.

He said, "I'm sorry, but you have prostate cancer." I had suspected it for some time. The biopsy was positive for cancer with a Gleason Score of 3 + 2, or 5. My doctor didn't bother to tell me what that meant. I found out later that the pathologists examine the cancer cells taken for the biopsy and give them a Gleason sum from 2 to 10, with 10 being very aggressive and dangerous. I was fortunate in that mine was about in the middle. (We will discuss PSA, biopsies, Gleason Grade and Stages in more detail in Chapter 6.)

BONE SCAN

He set up an appointment for me to have a bone scan. When prostate cancer starts spreading, it often goes into the bones. In a bone scan, the person is injected with radioactive material. The radioactive material will concentrate in a bone that has cancerous areas. If cancer is present in the bones it will show up as a dark "hot spot" on an X-ray.

It is a good test but totally unnecessary in about 90% in those cases where the PSA and Gleason Score are fairly low. Of course my bone scan was negative.

PROSTATECTOMY AND IMPOTENCE

It appeared that my cancer was localized. The doctor suggested that I have the prostate removed immediately. But I had heard about prostate surgery and impotence. I asked him what the chances were and he said about 50% of the men are usually impotent. The newer term is Erectile Dysfunction or ED.

Some men are never able to regain the ability to have an erection. This happens because the nerves that control the flow of blood into the penis, to cause an erection, may be severed or damaged. These nerves lie along the sides of the prostate. Until a few years ago, they were automatically removed along with the prostate.

In the early 1980s, physicians discovered that the erectile nerves can be peeled away from the prostate and preserved. The operation is a bit more difficult, and takes some time to learn. But an experienced doctor can remove the prostate and save the nerves and blood vessels, or neurovascular bundles. However, if it appears that the cancer has spread to the nerves usually the doctor will not try to save them. If only one side has been invaded, the nerve on the opposite side can often be saved so that erectile function can be preserved.

Some people may think that a 68-year-old man should not be too concerned about or interested in sex. I didn't feel like a 68-year-old man. When it came to sex, I felt just about the same as I did when I was 20 years old. It is true that I had slowed down a bit and I felt a few aches and pains now and then. But the pleasures of sex were every bit as good or better than they were 20 years ago. A 50% chance that I would no longer be able to enjoy sex was not the kind of odds that I wanted to chance.

SPERM BANKING

When you have a radical prostatectomy, you will still be able to have an orgasm, but you will never again be able to have an ejaculation. The seminal vesicles are removed along with the prostate. Even though your testes may still be producing millions of sperm, there is no way they can find their way out of the testes.

If you are a fairly young man and think that you may want to father a child at some later time, you might consider banking some of your sperm before you have a prostatectomy. Frozen sperm can last for several decades. Sperm from prize bulls has been frozen for over twenty years and is still viable. One bull has sired several thousand calves, even though he has been dead for several years.

Some doctors say that they are sometimes successful in taking sperm cells from the testes and using them to fertilize an ovum in vitro.

ALTERNATIVES TO PROSTATECTOMY

I asked my doctor about alternatives to surgery. He said it was possible to have radiation. Data shows that radiation is about as effective as surgery. More about surgery and radiation in later chapters.

He did offer one other alternative. I could do nothing. Some prostate cancers are relatively slow growing. I might be able to go for another five or six years before having the cancer treated. But then again some cancers may become very aggressive and begin growing and spreading very quickly. They can metastasize and spread beyond the prostate and throughout the body with little or no warning.

Other alternatives are radioactive seed implants and cryosurgery. In early 1992 these procedures were still new and considered to be experimental. These procedures are now recognized as viable treatments.

PROSTATE CANCER SUPPORT GROUPS

I made several phone calls and found that there are several Prostate Cancer support groups in the Los Angeles area. At one of the support group meetings, a medical doctor in his early 50s told about his prostate cancer. His prostate cancer had not been detected until it had spread throughout his body. A normal PSA for a man his age should be less than 4 nanograms per milliliter (4ng/ ml) of blood. His PSA was 524ng/ml.

You would think that a medical doctor would have known about his cancer before it had progressed so far. But it can be a silent killer that gives no real warning until it is too late. I talked with this doctor and he advised me to go ahead and have the operation before the cancer had a chance to spread. (This doctor underwent an experimental treatment with Suramin. More than nine years later, he is still alive and doing well. Another member of our support group had a PSA of 36. He also underwent the Suramin treatment at the same time and died three years later. The first rule when it comes to cancer is that there are no rules.)

After listening to the doctor's story and his advice, I decided to go ahead and have the prostatectomy. In the Bible, Ecclesiases, 9-4, it says, "Indeed, for any among the living there is hope; a live dog is better than a dead lion." I decided that I would be better off alive, and possibly impotent, than dead.

After being diagnosed in early January 1992, I made arrangements to have the operation done five months later in May of 1992.

THE PROSTATE OPERATION

On the day before my operation, I was given a couple of enemas and told to use them at night before I went to bed. I was not to have anything to eat after 11 P.M. The next day I checked into the hospital at 10 A.M. I was given several tests and signed several papers. At about 12:30 they gave me some tranquilizers and I drifted off to sleep.

I woke up at about 9 P.M. in the hospital after the operation. There were several cables going to a machine that was monitoring my heart and vital signs. There was an IV in the back of my left hand, an oxygen tube in my nose, a catheter, or Foley, in my penis and a catheter in the jugular vein of my neck. I found out later that I had required six units of blood.

Most doctors can do a prostatectomy with less than one unit of blood. Dr. E. David Crawford, one of the authors of this book, has done over 200 radical prostatectomies without having to give a transfusion.

EXPERIENCED DOCTORS

In the month before my operation, I gave two units of blood for my own use. They call this autologous blood. In these days of AIDS, and other blood-borne diseases, it is a good idea. Besides, the best blood for your body is your own.

Ordinarily, two units of blood should have been more than enough for the operation. The six units, or three liters, that I required was about half the blood in my entire body. An experienced doctor can do a prostatectomy in less than two hours. It took about five hours for my operation.

If you decide to have a prostatectomy, the first thing you should ask is how many such operations has the doctor performed. You should also ask about whether he does the nerve sparing operation. If the cancer is well contained, as mine was, most experienced doctors can remove the prostate without damaging the nerves that control erections. But if one bleeds as much as I did, there may be little chance to see the nerves and be able to preserve or spare them.

A new instrument from Uromed, called CaverMap, can help the surgeon identify the erectile nerves and preserve them. You can find out more about the CaverMap at www.uromed.com in Chapter Six.

Another new surgical tool that can help prevent blood loss is the LigaSure instrument. This instrument can be used to clamp off blood vessels, then using an electrical current, it divides and seals them. It is much easier, it is faster and seals much better than using a needle and catgut to ligate or tie off blood vessels. More about LigaSure in Chapter Six.

Before choosing a doctor, you should ask to talk with some of the patients that he has operated on. It is your life and your choice should be to get the best surgeon available. Don't worry about hurting the doctor's feelings. There is a tremendous difference in experience and skills among doctors. I didn't ask any of these questions. I am sorry that I didn't know enough then to ask them.

THE FOLEY CATHETER

During the operation, the prostate and the portion of the urethra that goes through the prostate are removed. The portion of the urethra below the prostate is pulled up and sewn to the bottom of the bladder neck. Before they do the operation, they insert a catheter, or rubber tube, up through the urethra of the penis into the bladder. The catheter is called a Foley.

The Foley has a small balloon on the bladder end. There is a small tube alongside of the main tube that allows them to inflate the balloon once the catheter is inside the bladder. The inflated balloon makes sure that the catheter cannot come out. The catheter allows the bladder to drain continuously while the cut portions of the urethra heal.

The catheter is attached to a plastic collection bag with a handle. On the third day I was able to get up and walk up and down the halls. Of course, I had to carry the plastic urine bag. The nurses teased me about carrying a purse. The bag does look a bit like a purse. But it is rather drab. I told them that the hospital should contact someone like Gucci and get a better design.

AT SIX DAYS

After six days in the hospital, they removed the stitches and I was allowed to return home. I was told to be very careful and not to exert myself in any way. They fitted me with a plastic urine bag that was strapped to my leg. In one respect, it was kind of nice. I never had to worry about getting up in the middle of the night to go potty.

Many patients are now encouraged to leave the hospital in less than two days. One of the largest expenses to an HMO is time spent in a hospital. I think they may have kept me longer because of the blood loss and operation difficulties.

A Reader's Digest had the account of a man who had prostate surgery in the early morning and was allowed to return home by noon. (It didn't say, but this was probably for BPH.) Dogs have prostates and have many of the same prostate problems that humans have. This guy took his beagle to the Vet for a prostate operation. The Vet said he would have to keep the dog overnight. The guy said, "That's strange. I went home after just four hours." The Vet said, "Yes, but your dog doesn't have an HMO."

AT TWO WEEKS

Two weeks after the operation I went back to my doctor for the removal of the Foley catheter. He deflated the balloon of the catheter and pulled it out. It wasn't much fun. My penis was very sore. I quickly learned that I had very little control over my bladder. Urine spurted out. The doctor had expected it and held an adult diaper around my penis to absorb the urine. He told me that it would be a while before I regained control of my bladder.

LEARNING TO URINATE

The doctor gave me instructions to do Kegel exercises. Kegel exercises strengthen the pelvic floor muscles. While urinating, I was instructed to stop and start the urine flow. Then try to determine which muscles I was using. I was then to practice contracting and relaxing these muscles several times each day. (We will discuss the Kegel exercise in more detail in Chapter 16 which deals with incontinence.)

THE REASON FOR INCONTINENCE

The prostate is intimately connected to the primary bladder valve that we use to control our urine. When they remove the prostate, they often remove part of the primary muscular valve or bladder sphincter. But we have a second muscular sphincter below the prostate that is usually left intact. It takes time, but with Kegel exercises, it can usually be trained to take over the job of controlling the urine.

ADULT DIAPERS

On the way home from the doctor's office I stopped and bought some adult diapers. Many women have incontinence problems, so most drugstores have several shelves stocked with two or more brands of the adult diapers.

The adult diapers are very similar to the leak-proof baby diapers. The diapers have a plastic outer liner and an absorbent material inside an inner liner. The inner material looks a bit like cotton, but when it becomes wet, it turns into a gel. It can hold quite a lot of water without ever leaking.

There are two main companies who manufacture most of the baby and adult diapers. Not long ago the two companies sued each other. Each company claimed that the other company had stolen their secret formula for the leak-proof diaper. The judge who heard the case had a great sense of humor. He said, "It appears that both of you have cases that hold water."

The first few days after the Foley was removed, I had very little control over my bladder, so I used a lot of diapers. A package of 36 diapers costs about $20. I finally got to where I regained a bit of control. I could stay dry for a couple of hours. But the minute I decided that I needed to go to the bathroom, it would start dribbling. Or if I sneezed, or exerted myself such as bending over it would dribble.

Of course I wore the diapers to bed. Usually I had no problems. But one night I felt a bit depressed. I had four or five glasses of wine before I went to bed. In the middle of the night I woke up in a pool of urine. The large amount of liquid was just too much for the diaper to absorb. I like wine very much, but after that I avoided having more than two glasses at night. I didn't have any more accidents, but just in case, I went down to the drugstore and bought some blue plastic liners that can be used on the bed to catch any urine.

I was able to wear the diapers under my street clothes so I could go out shopping, dining or whatever without any problems.

AT SIX WEEKS

At six weeks after the operation the soreness in my penis had pretty much disappeared. I tried several times to achieve an erection with no results. But I was able to achieve a sort of orgasm with vigorous stimulation and fantasy. (I still cannot say that I masturbated, because that is sinful and shameful, and something that nice people don't do.) The orgasm, if it can be called that, was not very satisfying. The pleasure and exhilaration of an ejaculation was missing. I was quite discouraged and very depressed.

AT NINE WEEKS

I had a checkup. My blood test for PSA was 0.2 or essentially non-detectable. It had been 10.2 before the operation. It appears that all of the cancer was removed. I felt very, very fortunate.

AT FOUR MONTHS

The doctor gave me a brief explanation about the drug papaverine. It is a vasodilator that dilates blood vessels that can cause an erection. It is a drug that is injected into the side of the penis. He gave me a prescription for the drug and syringes. The cost for the prescription and 100 needles was $70.00. I had it filled at a local pharmacy then returned to his office.

The first injection should be done under the supervision of the doctor. An ultra fine 29-gauge needle is used to inject the small amount of drug into the spongy body of the penis on one side. It immediately causes an influx of blood. The resulting erection may last for an hour or more.

Care must be taken that not too much is injected. It can possibly cause priapism, a prolonged erection that might require medical attention. Medicare will pay for several devices such as the vacuum devices and some of the penile implants and other procedures to combat impotence, but they will not pay for the papaverine drug. There are other drugs that have the same effect as papaverine. In 1995 the FDA approved the drug prostaglandin E1, the principle ingredient in Caverject, from the Upjohn Company for erectile dysfunction.

My doctor demonstrated how the drug should be administered. Since I am right handed, he had me grasp the head of my penis with my left hand, then had me wipe the right side of my penis with an alcohol-dampened tissue. He then handed me a filled syringe and told me to inject it into the side of my penis.

I don't like needles. I don't mind so much the needles involved in giving blood. I have given several gallons of blood. But I was very reluctant to have to stick a needle in my penis. I very nearly changed my mind. But I had gone without sex for so long that I was willing to try almost anything. I gritted my teeth and plunged the needle into my penis. Surprisingly, there was little or no pain. Within minutes my penis began to become erect. For the first time in many months, I had an erection.

I later learned that the drug is a mixture of papaverine and regitine which has a fairly short shelf life. Papaverine alone has a long shelf life, but when mixed with regitine and or prostaglandin, it should be refrigerated, much like the insulin drugs. The pharmacist should have told me this, but they don't handle this drug very often and just didn't know that much about it. I did not refrigerate it and sometime later I tried the drug and it didn't work. I was quite worried that there was something wrong with me.

It is critical that the drug be injected into a corpus cavernosum body of the penis. There is a corpus cavernosum body on each side of the penis. They are the bodies that are filled with blood to cause an erection. They both share blood vessels so you may inject on either side. If you miss the corpus cavernosum, there may be very little effect. Later I was able to buy an autoinjector. Just load the syringe into the autoinjector and press a button. It makes the injections much easier.

We will have more to say about papaverine, prostaglandin and other drugs and devices for impotence in Chapter 17 on erectile dysfunction and sex.

NINE MONTHS LATER, STILL IMPOTENT

At nine months I still could not achieve a normal erection. Several women friends have told me that it's not that important, that just being held and loved is enough. That just goes to show the vast difference between some men and women. Just being held and loved is great, but it's not enough for me.

I can still have orgasms even without an erection. Of course there is no ejaculate. There is a build up and a tension release but the orgasms are not quite as good as those I had before my operation. Perhaps I should say not the same, rather than not quite as good. Any time one can have an orgasm it is good. Woody Allen was quoted as saying that the worst sex he ever had was terrific. I have to agree.

Since I didn't have to manufacture an ejaculate, I should have been able to have several orgasms in a brief period. But alas, that was not the case.

I keep hoping that I will ultimately regain the ability to have normal erections. Doctors have said that it may take up to two years for the damaged nerves to regenerate and repair themselves.

AT TEN MONTHS

It has now been a little more than 10 months. Last night I woke up with a firm nocturnal erection. I was so excited that I could hardly go back to sleep. The next morning I figured that if I could get an erection while asleep, then I should be able to get one while awake. But no matter how hard I tried all I could manage was a semi or just half-hard erection. I am not sure now that I actually had an erection. Maybe I was just dreaming that I had the erection.

I have tried the vacuum erection devices (VED) and the injections. Both work, but the vacuum method is a bit uncomfortable. Poking a needle in the penis actually doesn't cause much pain, but still it is difficult to do. Besides, I still ooze urine when I try to have sex. So I use the vacuum device most of the time. It guarantees a good erection by drawing the blood into the penis, and then an elastic band is placed at the base of the penis. This elastic band constricts the venous outflow of blood to maintain the erection. This constriction also prevents the leakage of urine

AT ELEVEN MONTHS

I have awakened several more times with a nocturnal erection. But when I wake my lady friend and try to use it, it disappears almost immediately. I have since read that the physiological mechanism of a nocturnal erection is quite different than a normal erection. I still leak a lot of urine when I try to have sex. So I use the vacuum device with the rubber constriction ring.

I keep hoping that I will eventually regain the ability to have good erections. At a recent support group meeting one man proudly told everyone that he could achieve a normal erection about 70% of the time. I congratulated him and said that I can achieve a 50% erection about 70% of the time.

The literature defines three different stages to erection: flaccid, semi-rigid and rigid. In common terms, flaccid is soft and limp like a wet cooked noodle. Some of the men in our group have talked about trying to have sex with the limp wet noodle. Semi-rigid is half-hard or half-mast. With a lot of cooperation and help from your partner, it is possible to have sex with a semi-rigid penis. Some call this a "stuffer" type erection because it can be stuffed into a willing vagina with a little help.

Rigid is the goal that most of us hope for. But for me, and a lot of others, it may be as difficult to achieve as finding the pot of gold at the end of a rainbow.

My latest PSA was still undetectable.

AT 13 MONTHS

I still awake sometimes at night with a nocturnal erection, but I have noticed that my penis has a distinct curve when erect. I still cannot have a normal erection. I still use the VED and penile injections. The curve is not very evident when I have an erection by using the VED. But it is quite pronounced when I have an erection due to the injection.

It appears that I might have a slight case of Peyronie's Disease. In this disease, fibrosis sets up in some of the tissue layers, usually on the top or bottom of the penis. The area becomes hard and inelastic so that during an erection, the penis is bent because the side that has the disorder cannot expand. If the disease is on the top of the penis, it will be bent upwards. This may not cause too much of a problem. When it bends downward such as mine does, I was not able to have sex with the injections. I can still have sex by using the VED. But even then, it is a bit painful.

I am quite unhappy and depressed. After the prostate cancer and not being able to have normal erections, I now have this disease. I would cry if I thought it would help. I found out later that many men may have slight curvatures, up down, left or right without having Peyronie's disease. It may not cause much of a problem unless it is severely bent.

AT 14 MONTHS

I still wake up at night with firm nocturnal erections. When I feel it, there is the pronounced downward bend in the middle at almost a 45-degree angle. This is due to the onset of Peyronie's disease. When I use the Osbon VED there is still a downward bend. The downward bend is even more pronounced with the injections and makes it impossible to have sex. If it gets much worse I may have to have surgery. In the meantime, my urologist suggested that I take a lot of vitamin E.

Usually I take multivitamins and a 400 unit vitamin E. I began taking 400 units of vitamin E three times a day. I also used my VED to help straighten out the curvature in my penis. I am not sure it would work for everyone, but it definitely helped me. After 6 months of the high dose vitamin E and the VED, I still have a bit of curvature, but it does not cause any problems.

AT 24 MONTHS

It has now been over two years since my operation. I still am unable to have a normal erection. I am still using the injections. They work well but I still have urine leakage when I use it.

The urine leakage can be a real problem at times. Quite often when I see a beautiful woman, I start fantasizing. Of course this starts the urine leakage. So there are times when I can't even have a decent fantasy, let alone doing the real thing. But in spite of all these unfortunate things, I am still very fortunate compared to some men.

When I give myself an injection, I am ready almost immediately. I mentioned to my lady friend that perhaps the drug companies should devise a similar drug for women. Just think of all the foreplay time that could be saved. She didn't think it was funny. I was just kidding of course, I enjoy foreplay. Female sexual dysfunction can be a real problem. Several companies are now developing drugs and devices to help them overcome it.

AT THREE YEARS

The Peyronie's has almost completely healed. I still have a small amount of curvature, but it does not cause any problem. I have taken a lot of vitamin E over the last two years and used my vacuum device a lot. I don't know for sure, but I think it helped. I am still impotent. I participated in the study using the prostaglandin E1 for over a year.

My PSA is still less than 0.1 ng/ml. For most standard PSA tests, 0.1 and 0.2 are considered undetectable. I have every expectation that it will remain at this level over the next two years.

AT NINE YEARS

At the present time of this revision, in 2001, I am still impotent, or rather I have Erectile Dysfunction (ED), the accepted term today. I still use my vacuum device. I have worn out two pumps but they were replaced by Osbon at no charge. They give a lifetime guarantee on the major components. (Call Osbon at 1-800-438-8592 for a copy of an informative booklet and a brochure about their ErecAid. They also have a web site at http://www.timmmedical.com/ . The web site has photos and a vast amount of information about the VED).

I am also still using the injections. I tried MUSE, which is prostaglandin E1 (PGE1), the same drug that is used in the injections. It is a pellet that is inserted into the urethra. It has to be absorbed through the urethral tissues, and even at 1000 micrograms, it is not as effective as 10 micrograms of PGE1 when injected. The body is very good at preventing any foreign agent from penetrating the skin or even the urethra. The VIVUS Company is re-formulating MUSE and it is expected to be much more effective.

In order for Viagra to be effective, you must have the erectile nerves. Since my nerves were severed, Viagra helps to give me only a partial erection. I take Viagra, then use my vacuum device to create a rigid erection.

I still have a leakage of urine, but it is not quite as bad as in the beginning.

The reason for the urine leakage is quite simple. Before my prostatectomy, I would often wake up in the morning with an erection or pee hard-on. When I tried to urinate, it was very difficult. The reason is that the bladder sphincter, or valve, automatically closes tightly when a man has an erection. This is done so that the semen will be forced out of the penis during ejaculation rather than taking the shorter route to the bladder.

The prostate is an intimate part of the bladder valve. When cutting the prostate away, the primary sphincter or bladder valve, is often damaged. But fortunately, we have a second musculo-membraneous valve below the prostate. By doing Kegel exercises this valve can be trained to take over the function of the original bladder valve.

But all of my life, this secondary valve opened when I had an erection in order to let the semen out. So even when I try to have an erection, it automatically opens. Of course it lets the urine out. Even if I empty my bladder before trying to have sex, there seems to always be a bit of urine there.

In spite of the urine and ED problems, I still feel fortunate in that my PSA is still undetectable. I am much better off than many, many men. My urine problem pales when compared to some men whose secondary valve was also destroyed. These men have no control over their urine at all. The only answer for some of them is to have an artificial urinary sphincter (AUS) installed. More about incontinence in Chapter 1.

When I consider what the men who are on CHT, or worse yet chemotherapy, have to endure, my problems are very minor. I feel very, very fortunate. At least I am still alive and can expect to live for another 15 years or so if I don't get killed on the Los Angeles freeways or in an earthquake.

Chapter Four

THE PROSTATE, PENIS AND REPRODUCTIVE SYSTEM

Dr. Aubrey Pilgrim

The male reproductive system is made up of the testes, the vas deferens, the seminal vesicles, the prostate and the penis. See fig. 4-1. At the onset of puberty in the male, testosterone causes the testes to start manufacturing sperm cells. In the female, estrogen causes the breasts to enlarge and the ovaries to start maturing and releasing ova cells.

THE CREATION OF SPERM AND OVA CELLS

Chromosomes are strands of DNA in the nucleus of cells that carries all of the genes. Each of the several hundred trillion cells in a person's body has 23 pairs of chromosomes except for the sperm cells in males and ova cells in females. The infantile sperm and ova cells start out with 23 pairs of chromosomes just like all of the other cells in the body. But they go through a special process of division, called meiosis, so that each sperm and each ovum ends up with only 23 single chromosomes. When a lucky little sperm combines with an ovum it completes the 23 pairs of chromosomes.

The 23rd chromosome in the sperm cell is either an X or Y chromosome. About half the sperm will have an X chromosome, the other half will have a Y. The female ova all have an X chromosome. The X and Y chromosomes from the male determines sex. If a sperm cell with an X chromosome fertilizes an egg it combines with the X chromosome of the ovum to produce a female. If a sperm cell with a Y chromosome enters an egg it will produce a male (Y =Boy).

Incidentally, a female is born with all of the egg cells she will ever have, about 400,000. Most women have a fertile period of about 30 years. After puberty, normally one egg per month ripens and drops. So most women will only drop from 360 to 400 eggs in their lifetime. Nowadays, most women only have two or three children in their lifetime so most of the eggs that do mature and drop are flushed away.

A normal young male produces about 250 million sperm for each ejaculation. A young male may be able to ejaculate three or more times in a single day.

THE VAS DEFERENS

After the sperm cells go through meiosis, they move into the epididymis area of the testes to finish maturation. The vas deferens are two tubes that connects the epididymis and the seminal vesicles. During ejaculation, the tubular musculature of the vas deferens constricts and forces the sperm up into the prostate. The prostate and seminal vesicles add the milky gelatinous substance to the sperm cells, then the prostate squeezes down and forces the ejaculate out through the urethra. The ejaculatory ducts enter the prostate from the back at a 45 degree angle and empty into the urethra.

Of course, several other organs, nerves and muscles, also contribute to an orgasm and ejaculation.

The vas deferens tubes lie very close to the surface just below the penis. When a vasectomy is done, they make a small slit in the skin between the penis and the testicles and lift the vas deferens out. The two tubes are then tied off, or ligated, in two places. The tubes are then severed between the ligations. It is a very simple operation and fairly painless.

VASECTOMY AND PROSTATE CANCER

A February 17, 1993 issue of the Journal of the American Medical Association (JAMA) had two studies of the effects of vasectomies on men and risk of prostate cancer. According to the authors of this study, the risk varied from 56 percent greater to as much 89 percent for men who had a vasectomy 20 years or more earlier.

In the same issue there was an editorial that questioned the study and the vasectomy-prostate cancer link. They cited other studies that did not show such a link. The editors suggested that there was little reason for alarm. But they did suggest that men who have had vasectomies should get an annual DRE and PSA test. Vasectomy or not, that is good advice for all men over 50. That is the same advice that the American Urologic Association (AUA) and the American Cancer Society (ACS) has preached for some time.

Most urologists believe that the study was severely flawed and that a man who has a vasectomy has no greater risk of prostate cancer than any other man. It did appear that men who had undergone a vasectomy were diagnosed with prostate cancer more often than men who had not had a vasectomy. It is believed that the reason may be that a man who has had a vasectomy is usually more concerned about his health and therefore may have checkups more often.

If you are considering having a vasectomy, or treatments for prostate cancer, and you think that you may want to father children later, then maybe you should have some of your sperm frozen. Frozen sperm can last for many years.

One other advantage of having a vasectomy is that it can make a great conversation subject. My wife and I went to many parties in our younger days. I would often find a pretty girl and when we ran out of something to talk about, I would offer to show her my vasectomy scars. But my wife was usually hovering nearby, so I never got the chance.

THE DIFFERENCE IN PROSTRATE AND PROSTATE

You won't hear anyone who has had prostate cancer make the mistake, but some people confuse the word prostrate and prostate. The word prostrate is from the Latin *prostratus* which means to cast down. It usually means to lie face down.

The word prostate is from the Greek *prostates*, which means one who stands before. I have no idea why they called it that. It may be because if you start at the end of the penis and go up the urethra, it stands before you get to the bladder.

GROWTH AND DEVELOPMENT OF THE PROSTATE

In a young male baby, the prostate is about the size of a green pea. It gradually increases in size until puberty, then there is a rapid growth until the person is about 30 years old. The normal prostate of a 30-year-old man weighs about 20 grams or ¾ of an ounce and is about the size of a chestnut. It fact, it is shaped a bit like a chestnut.

It normally stays about 20 grams until the man reaches about 45 years old, then quite often, it begins to increase in size. Some have suggested that this spurt of growth may be associated with a "male menopause". No one knows for sure the reason for the extra growth.

SIMILARITIES OF THE PROSTATE AND THE BREAST

Prostate cancer is the leading cancer in men, breast cancer is the leading cancer in women. The number of women who are diagnosed with breast cancer is about the same as the number of men who are diagnosed with prostate cancer. About 42,000 women die from breast cancer each year, about 30,000 to 40,000 men die from prostate cancer.

Another similarity is that both prostate and breast tissue are hormone sensitive. According to Dr. Jacob Rajfer of UCLA, if a young boy is given testosterone before puberty, his prostate will become enlarged. His penis will also become larger and longer. If a young girl is given estrogen before puberty, her breasts will develop and become larger.

If a man is given testosterone after puberty, his prostate will become larger, but his penis will not get any bigger, no matter how much testosterone he is given. If a woman is given estrogen after puberty, her breasts will not grow any larger. But if a man is given estrogenic hormones it will cause his breasts to become enlarged. Some of the hormones used for treatment of advanced prostate cancer are similar to female hormones. One of the side effects of these treatments is gynecomastia, or breast enlargement. Some men are so embarrassed that they resort to having breast reduction surgery.

PELVIC TISSUES AND STRUCTURES

Though the normal prostate is a fairly small gland, it may grow quite large. This may be especially so in some older men who develop Benign Prostatic Hyperplasia (BPH). Instead of being the size of a chestnut, some may grow as large as an orange or larger. (More about BPH in the next chapter.)

Besides being a cancer site, the prostate may be the site of several other problems such as prostatitis, (the suffix—*itis* means inflammation), prostadynia (the suffix—*dynia* means pain), prostatic calculi or stones, and benign prostatic hyperplasia (BPH). Prostatitis and prostadynia may be caused by bacterial infection, calcification of small stones or a number of other causes.

The prostate is very much a part of, and involved in, many of the pelvic tissues. The prostate can cause you a lot of trouble. It can even kill you. To paraphrase John Dunne, no prostate is an island entire unto itself, for it is involved in all pelvic tissues. Several organs and tissues in the pelvic region are intimately connected or related to the prostate. When the prostate is affected by disease or cancer, many of these closely related organs and tissues are also affected.

THE BLADDER SPHINCTER

The sphincter vesicae is a circular muscle around the neck of the bladder. It is the urethral valve that we use to control our urine when we void or pee. Ordinarily, this muscular valve is in a state of constriction at all times except when we urinate. When we need to urinate, a signal is sent through the nervous system from the brain down to the sphincter muscles. The sphincter opens and allows the bladder to empty. The urine passes through the urinary canal, or urethra, through the center of the prostate and out of the penis.

The circular muscular fibers of the bladder sphincter are continuous with the muscular fibers of the prostate. Since the prostate and the sphincter vesicae are so intimately connected, some of the circular muscles of the bladder sphincter are often removed or damaged during a radical prostatectomy. After the prostate is removed, the bladder is pulled down and the cut ends of the urethra are sewn to the bladder.

THE PROSTATE

The prostate is an integral part of the male reproductive system. It is located just below the urinary bladder. It looks a bit like a small apple that is somewhat flattened. Usually we think of the base of an object being at the bottom and the apex being at the top. But the larger top portion of the prostate is called the base and the smaller bottom portion is called the apex.

The base blends into the circular muscles of the bladder sphincter or urinary valve which connects to the urethra. The apex is connected to the musculo membraneous urethra sphincter or the external striated urethral sphincter. This is the sphincter that many men have to train with Kegels after a prostatectomy.

The front or anterior portion of the prostate is directly behind the pubic bone. The back portion or peripheral zone contacts the outer layer of the rectal tube. When a doctor puts his gloved finger in the rectum, he can usually feel any abnormalities through the rectal wall.

In performing a DRE an experienced doctor can get a good estimate of the size of the prostate and whether it is enlarged or not. The doctor can also feel the consistency. It should be smooth, soft and uniform. Ordinarily, most cells have spaces around them that are filled with lymphatic fluid. Tumors are usually packed very tightly and close together so that they are hard and lumpy. If there are any unusual lumps or nodules or if it is hard and grainy, it will be cause for suspicion of cancer.

The front portion of the prostate is directly behind the pubic bone so it cannot be palpated. Most prostate cancers arise in the rear peripheral zone of the prostate so they can be easily palpated or felt through the rectal wall. Of course those that arise in the middle zones may not be detected by a DRE unless the tumor is very large. That is why the PSA and ultra sound are such important diagnostic tools. A DRE, ultrasound and a PSA blood test can detect most all prostate cancer.

The prostate is enveloped by a thin fibrous capsule. In prostate cancer stages T1 and T2 the cancer will be entirely within the capsule. In T3 stages, it will have broken through the capsule. It may have sent out branches that infiltrated some of the local pelvic tissues and organs. In T4 stages, it has broken through the capsule and metastasized. Cancer cells may have escaped through the blood or lymph system to distant areas of the body where new colonies have set up.

In the older Whitmore-Jewett system of staging, we used the letters A, B, C and D. The newer Tumor-Node-Metastasis (TNM) system is much more descriptive of the stages. More about diagnosis and staging systems in Chapter Six.

THE MALE UTERUS

You will find just about everything in a man that you will find in a woman and vice versa. (Only the things look much better on a woman.) The prostatic utricle is a small pouch or cul-de-sac located in the central portion of the prostatic urethra. It is called by some the uterus masculinus, or male uterus. It may also be called the Mullerian Duct. The male uterus is about 6 millimeters long or about one fourth of an inch. The October 1992 issue of Urology Journal reported a case of cancer in the prostatic utricle or Mullerian Duct. The man had uterine cancer.

THE FEMALE PROSTATE GLAND

Again, both males and females have similar organs, glands and structures. In many, the organ in the opposite sex may be only rudimentary, but it is there nonetheless. My old Gray's Anatomy, says that the "Skene's ducts in the female urethra are regarded as the homologues of the prostatic glands".

Taber's Cyclopedic Medical dictionary, says that Skene's glands lie "just inside of and on the posterior of the urethra in the female." This means that they are just beneath the bladder, in the same general location as the prostate gland in men.

Dr. Judith Brumm, one of the few female urologists, said that she had a woman patient who had cancer in her Skene's glands.

This was essentially prostate cancer.

The G spot in the vagina is in the Skene's glands. The G spot was named for Dr. Ernst Grafenberg who discovered it in 1950. It is located about an inch inside the vagina, in the top portion, behind the pubic bone. When stimulated in most women, the area swells and may become about the size of a half-dollar. It may feel a bit spongy. For many women, stimulating the G spot can cause them to have an intense orgasm.

The prostate in most men continues to grow and enlarge, especially in older men. This is benign prostatic hyperplasia (BPH). One reason for the continued growth is testosterone. Since the Skene's glands are not subjected to testosterone, they do not become enlarged with age such as the prostate does. Just as in men, these glands are subject to sexually transmitted diseases such as gonorrhea.

THE EJACULATE

When a man is sexually aroused and ejaculates, sperm travels from the testicles through the two vas deferens tubes to the seminal vesicles, then through the prostate to empty into the urethra, then out of the penis. There are usually from 60 million to 250 million sperm in each ejaculation.

During ejaculation, seminal fluid is added as the sperm pass through the seminal vesicles. The seminal fluid is made up of fructose (sugar), zinc and other minerals. As the sperm passes through the prostate, an acidic prostatic fluid is added along with PSA. Even though there may be 250 million sperm cells, they are very tiny. It would take about 600 of them, laid end to end to equal one inch.

The prostate is made up of muscles and hundreds of small glands. The glands manufacture the milky fluid that is mixed with the semen and sperm cells during ejaculation. About 95% of the bulk of the ejaculate is made up of prostatic and seminal fluid. The prostatic fluid and the semen provide nutrition and a swimming medium for the sperm cells.

The prostate normally produces a small amount of PSA which is mixed with the ejaculate. The ejaculate is a thick opalescent gel. The PSA causes the ejaculate to become liquefied which makes it easier for the sperm to swim in.

The total volume for a normal ejaculation is from 2.0 mL to 5.0 mL. (5.0 mL is equal to one teaspoon). As men get older, the volume will be less. If a man has had a radiation treatments or seed implants, he may have a much lessened ejaculate or possibly, no ejaculate at all. If he has had a radical prostatectomy, he will not have any ejaculate at all, or possibly a small amount of fluid from the Cowper's glands

The seminal vesicles are two membranous pouches behind the bladder and in front of the rectum. The seminal vesicles contribute a portion of the ejaculate.

During sexual arousal, the prostate manufactures a large amount of prostatic fluid. Some of the fluid is usually forced out of the penis before ejaculation. This helps to lubricate the urethra for the passage of the ejaculate.

During ejaculation, the muscles of the prostate gland, the seminal vesicles and the vas deferens all act in unison to contract, squeeze and propel the ejaculate out of the penis. (I once heard a question asked, how far can a man ejaculate? Someone answered, about 5000 feet if he is standing on the bank of the Grand Canyon. Actually it is only a few inches, depending primarily on the age of the man.)

The contraction of the muscles of the vas deferens, the seminal vesicles and the prostate gland adds to the sensation of orgasm. After a prostatectomy, a man can still have an orgasm, but he may not have the same sensation without the contraction of the prostate gland and seminal vesicles.

Because of their intimate connection with the prostate, it is possible that the seminal vesicles could be infiltrated with cancer cells. They are nearly always removed during a prostatectomy. Besides, with the removal of the prostate, there is no way that the seminal vesicles could empty the semen and sperm into the urethra.

ERECTION NERVES

The prostate is richly endowed with veins, arteries and nerves. Branches of the nerves and blood vessels that supply the prostate are also the primary nerves and blood vessels that supply the penis. In the early days, when a surgeon removed the prostate, all of the nerves and blood vessels near it were also removed. The removal of these nerves and blood vessels meant that the man would be impotent for the rest of his life and would never be able to have a normal erection.

In the early 1980s, investigators identified the nerve bundles, branches and blood vessels that supplied the penis. They found that these neurovascular bundles could be peeled them away from the prostate and left intact. Main branches of these nerves and blood vessels are on both sides of the prostate.

During a radical prostatectomy, if it appears that the cancer is only on one side of the prostate, that neurovascular bundle can be widely excised. If the other side appears to be free of cancer, that side can be left undamaged. With one side of the nerves preserved the odds of remaining potent is fairly good.

Of course, if there is a chance that the cancer is involved in the nerves and blood vessels on both sides, they would be excised. Depending on the age and past sexual history of the patient, with intact nerves, up to 75% of younger patients may regain potency within a year or so. Up to 90% of patients may regain potency when helped by Viagra.

The CaverMap is an electronic device that can help the surgeons identify and preserve the erectile nerves.

THE MEMBRANOUS URETHRAL SPHINCTER

Just below the prostate is another circular bundle of muscles that form the membranous urethral sphincter. This muscle is also found in women.

Normally the bladder sphincter and the membranous sphincter are closed. During micturition (a nice word that means to pee or urinate), both sphincters relax to allow the passage of urine. At the end of urination, the bladder sphincter closes and the membranous sphincter is then used to squeeze out the last few drops.

Again, the bladder sphincter is often damaged during a radical prostatectomy. We are fortunate in that the musculo-membranous urethral sphincter below the prostate can be trained to take over the job of the primary bladder sphincter. The membranous urethral sphincter is more easily trained to perform this function in some men than in others. Some men can be dry in a matter of two or three months. It may take others up to a year or more. In some men, the membranous urethral sphincter may have been damaged along with the primary bladder sphincter. Because of this and other causes, a small percentage of men may never regain urinary control.

COWPER'S GLANDS

If you have had a prostatectomy, you may be surprised to find that you still have a small discharge during sexual arousal. The viscous fluid that is seen is from the Cowper's glands, also called the bulbourethral glands. They are two small glands within the lower portion of the urethra. They are about the size of peas. They each have a duct that opens into the urethra. The small amount of fluid they manufacture is similar to the prostatic fluids or ejaculate.

Cowper's glands are very unique and puzzling. Dr. Donald Coffey has pointed out that the Cowper's glands are made up of the same type of cells and tissues as the prostate, yet there has never been a case of cancer found in these glands.

There is another puzzling aspect of the Cowper's glands. As men grow older, the prostate gland increases in size; but the similar tissues in Cowper's glands diminish in size with age.

Women have two small Bartholin glands near the vaginal opening at the base of the labia majora that are homologues of the male Cowper's glands. During sexual arousal, women may also have a small discharge from their Bartholin glands that is similar to the discharge produced by the Cowper's glands in males. Dr. Coffey didn't say so, but women probably do not get cancer in their Bartholin glands.

THE PELVIS

The pelvis is made of large bones, shaped somewhat like a bowl. The two large hip bones are called ilia, which is Latin for groins or flanks. The ilia are connected to the sacrum and tail bone in the back. The femur heads, or ball sections, of the leg bones attach to the sockets of the hip bones. The lower part of the hip bones are called ischia, which is Greek for hip. The pubic bones meet and join in the front.

The bottom part of the pelvic girdle is called the pelvic floor. Several muscles and ligaments make up the floor. The rectum, the urethra and corpora cavernosa of the penis all pass through the pelvic floor. One reason it is so difficult to do a prostatectomy is that it is completely surrounded by the pelvic bones.

THE PENIS

The penis is composed of three cylindrical bodies of cavernous tissue. (Cavernous means that it has hollow spaces.) Two of the bodies, the left corpus cavernosum and the right corpus cavernosum, lie along side each other. The third body, the corpus spongiosum houses the urethra and is located beneath the two corpora cavernosa. See fig. 4-2. The cavernosus bodies, or corpora cavernosa, are the spongy bodies that fill with blood to form an erection. At the external end of the three bodies is the glans penis or the head. (*Glans* is Latin for acorn, which somewhat describes the shape of the head of the penis.)

The entire penis is covered by a loose skin. The head of the penis is covered by the foreskin which is removed if the person has been circumcised. (I went to a party recently. A woman asked me, "What do you call that superfluous skin around a penis?" Before I could answer she said, "A man." Some women have a twisted sense of humor. I didn't think it was funny at all.)

About one third of the penis is inside the body and extends most of the way back to the anus. The bulbocavernosus muscle is wrapped around this portion of the penis. (The prefix *bulb* in bulbocavernosus is from Latin bulbous meaning root). It can constrict the urethra and help empty it after urination. The bulbocavernosus helps during an erection by compressing the deep dorsal vein of the penis, thus trapping the blood to help maintain the erection.

The ischiocavernosus muscles are attached to, and wrap around the penis. There are branches of the muscle on each side which extend backward and attach to the inside of the pelvis near the inner part of the hip socket. These muscles also help in achieving an erection by compression of the veins that exit the cavernosus bodies. These muscles help to anchor and tie the penis to the inside of the pelvic bones. During an ejaculation or orgasm, these muscles contract rhythmically and contribute to the pleasant sensation.

From its origin in the back near the anus, the penis curves upward and is anchored in the front of the body to the pubic bone by suspensory ligaments. See fig. 4-1. In operations for penile augmentation and lengthening, these suspensory ligaments are severed. Severing these ligaments may add up to one inch to the length of the penis.

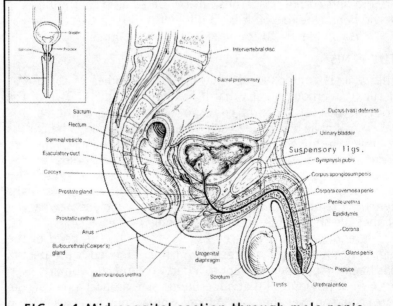

FIG. 4-1 Mid-saggital section through male penis. (Courtesy Zeneca Corp.)

The clitoris is a rudimentary penis. It may be four inches or more long internally and have equivalent attachments as a penis.

CONTROL OF CIRCULATION BY THE NERVOUS SYSTEM

You probably know that the arteries carry oxygen and other nutrients to the various tissues. It gives up the oxygen and nutrition, then picks up the carbon dioxide and other wastes. It moves through the capillaries into the veins and back to the heart to be circulated again.

The blood vessels are actually round muscular tubes. The body regulates its blood pressure by causing the musculature around some arteries to constrict while relaxing others. If a person has just eaten a large meal, lots of blood is needed in the abdominal area to help digest it. The arteries are relaxed in the abdomen so that more blood is available. But we have a closed system, so some of the blood vessels in other areas must be constricted and made smaller in order to force more blood into the abdominal area. This regulation is done automatically by the nervous system.

WHAT CAUSES AN ERECTION

I know a lady who is a school nurse. Part of her job is to give a lecture to the 5th and 6th grade boys about their developing bodies and puberty. In one of these classes she explained that boys may sometimes have nocturnal erections. Then she explained how the influx of blood into the penis could cause an erection. She noticed that one boy, who seemed to be a bit older than the others, wasn't

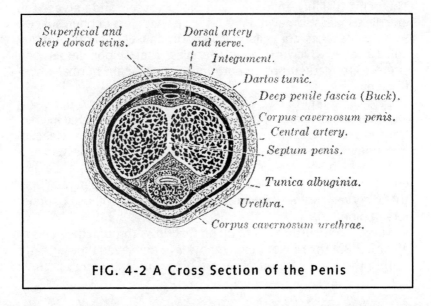

FIG. 4-2 A Cross Section of the Penis

paying much attention. She asked him if he could repeat to the class what caused an erection. He said, "Sure. Thinking about pretty girls."

That used to do it for me, but since I have had my prostatectomy, it just doesn't work any more. An erection requires that the brain, nerves, heart, blood vessels and hormones all work together. It may also require, especially as we get older, a bit of visual stimulation and a bit of plain old manual stimulation.

We have in our body three different types of muscles; skeletal muscles such as those of the arms and legs, smooth muscles such as those of the intestines and blood vessels and the cardiac or heart muscle. We also have the central nerve systems which includes the brain and spinal cord and the somatic or peripheral nerve system.

The peripheral nerve system includes those that are under our direct conscious control such as those used to cause an arm or leg to move. We also have an autonomic or involuntary nerve system that causes many of our body's system to work automatically. We have no conscious control over the autonomic system.

The autonomic system has two types of nerves, the sympathetic and the parasympathetic. The two systems act to keep each other in balance. An analogy would be an automobile, which has an accelerator to make it move and a brake to stop it. The sympathetic and parasympathetic nervous systems control the blood vessels that cause erections.

Most of the tissue that forms the penis is called erectile tissue. The penis is richly endowed with blood vessels and nerves. The erectile tissue is somewhat like a sponge with lots of open spaces. The open spaces are called lacunae or sinuses. There are many small arteries which are called arterioles. These blood vessels and sinuses are made up of smooth muscle which are normally contracted.

Dr. Jacob Rajfer of UCLA found that when a man becomes sexually aroused, the parasympathetic nerves that are involved in erections cause certain chemicals such as nitric oxide to be released. The body also produces a chemical called phosphodiesterase 5 (PDE5) which acts to keep the penile blood vessels in a state of contraction. Viagra is a PDE5 inhibitor. Along with the parasympathetic nerves and nitric oxide, the blood vessels will relax and let lots of blood in.

There is a small amount of blood that flows through the penis at all times. But the rate of blood inflow is about seven times greater during the state of arousal. There are veins and venules (small veins) in the penis which normally carry blood away. Enclosing the penis, just beneath the skin, is a tough fibrous sheath, the tunica albuginea. At the same time that the penile arteries are relaxing and filling the sinuses, the erection causes the veins to be compressed against the tunica albuginea. Since there is no way out for the arterial blood, the penis becomes erect and ready for action. The erection remains until the sympathetic nerves cause the arteries to become constricted and the nitric oxide is no longer produced. If the parasympathetic nerves are severed or damaged during a radical prostatectomy, there will be no production of nitric oxide and Viagra will have little or no effect.

There are several causes of impotence or erectile dysfunction. Urologists have found that some men who are impotent may have penile veins that do not become constricted to keep the arterial blood in the penis. This allows the blood to leak out almost as fast as it comes in. There are other cases where there may be arterial insufficiency and not enough blood can be pumped in. There may be several different reasons for this such as an obstruction caused by atherosclerosis or hardening of the arteries. Some of these afflictions may be helped with microsurgery.

Smoking and several drugs can also interfere with the erection process. Some of the several causes of erectile dysfunction will be discussed in Chapter 17.

STUDYING THE PENIS

Scientists are now devoting more time and resources to the study of the penis. Almost every issue of the Journal of Urology has at least one article on these different studies. Some of the studies involve testing drugs such as papaverine, phentolamine, and prostaglandins. (The drug prostaglandin was first discovered in the prostate gland, thus the name.) These drugs are vasodilators. When injected into the penis they can cause erections.

If the drugs are administered in a laboratory setting, it is quite different than being in a private room and having a waiting and willing partner. So the injections may not always work in the laboratory. To try to overcome this problem, one study had the participants view an X-rated porno tape along with the drugs. They called this adjunct to the protocol visual sexual stimulation (VSS). They wanted to see if the tapes improved the effectiveness of the drugs. But many people still have a lot of Judeo-Christian feelings of guilt and sinfulness about anything as personal as the penis. Some of the men in this test were outraged over the porno tapes and withdrew from the experiment.

Even those men who have no religious beliefs may be uncomfortable with some of the needed experiments and tests. Some tests may require that several experimenters observe and perform measurements while the man tries to get an erection. Not many men can perform under these circumstances. Usually it is a male doctor of urology or an andrologist who does the testing on men. (*Andro* is a prefix for man; *gyne* means woman, so an andrologist for men is somewhat comparable to a gynecologist for women.)

A friend was is in a clinical trial for testing the penile injections. He had a pretty nurse who observed and measured his penis for length and girth. She checked him frequently for tumescence or hardness by squeezing his penis while testing the drug. This was definitely better than the VSS protocol. One of the goals of clinical trials is to test the efficacy of the drugs on a person who is truly impotent. If a man does not get an erection while a pretty woman manipulates his penis, then he is probably impotent.

One test often used in the trials is to have the man stand, then the doctor or nurse uses a compass to measure the degree of the angle of the penis at various times. Before my operation, I had no trouble attaining a 45 degree upward angle. Even with the injection to cause an erection, the best I can do now is about five degrees downward. This may have been a side effect of my radical prostatectomy.

Another test is to use a gauge that is pressed against the head of the penis. This measures the rigidity of the erect penis. The gauge can measure how much pressure can be applied before the penis buckles or bends. There are other sophisticated gauges such as the rigiscan that can measure the rigidity of the penis.

Because of laboratory limitations, many scientists use rats, rabbits, dogs and other animals for experimentation. They can perform experiments on these animals that would be impossible on a human being. They often test drugs by injecting them into the penis of a mouse. Can you imagine the difficulty in relating tests done on the penis of a mouse to the penis of a man? Can you imagine injecting the penis of a mouse to cause him to get an erection?

Dogs are often used in penile studies because they have a larger penis. They also have a prostate. One study that was reported in a Urology Journal involved the problem of retrograde ejaculation. This often happens to a man after undergoing a transurethral prostatectomy (TURP) for an enlarged prostate. The primary bladder sphincter valve is often damaged so that it does not close completely during ejaculation. So at ejaculation, the sperm will take the shorter path and go into the bladder.

A prostate operation similar to a TURP was performed on the dogs. After the dogs had healed they masturbated the dogs to check for retrograde ejaculation. They were able to study the dogs in ways that would never be possible with a man.

PENILE AUGMENTATION

In the Declaration of Independence, Thomas Jefferson wrote..."We hold these truths to be self evident, that all men are created equal..." You were wrong, Mr. Jefferson. Not all men or all women are created equal. Some are born beautiful, with all of the luxuries that life can possibly afford. Many more are born poor, homely, obese, diseased and destined to endure humiliation and suffering all of their lives.

Even if they don't have these adverse afflictions, many men and women are unhappy with their bodies. They are usually too fat, too short or too tall or bald. Many women are usually unhappy with the size of their breasts; the men with the size of their penises.

Women can have breast implants that can instantly give them any endowment they desire. Many comedians made a career of telling jokes about breasts. I even got on the bandwagon myself back in 1960s with this line:

Not A Laughing Matter

Mammoplastic augmentation
Is no cause for titillation.

Psychologists and common sense tell us that the size of the breasts should not make any difference in the enjoyment of sex. (As far as I know, man is the only mammal who considers the mammary glands to be linked to sex. To other mammals, the size and shape of the mammary glands has nothing to do with sex). But our ideals of what is beautiful and desirable goes back a long way. Look at some of the ancient sculptures and paintings. So who can blame a woman for wanting to look her best and most desirable if that is what men want.

"It's too big" are three little words that most men will never hear from a woman. The average length of the adult male erect penis is about five inches. If you have seen X-rated movies, you know that there are a few men who may have been born with an endowment that is a lot more than average. There are probably many more men who are unhappy with the size of their penis than women with the size of their breasts.

I attended a presentation on impotence treatments using injections at a recent AUA Convention. A doctor stated that a long penis was subject to buckling and being rather limp. The doctor said that a short penis responded much better to injections and usually resulted in an erection that was much more rigid and firm. That may be true, but there probably isn't a man alive, with the possible exception of the Pope, who would not like to be longer.

A lot of men are so concerned about penis size that they have had penile augmentation. Most of them could have saved the money because they were probably normal to begin with. What's "Normal"? Well, it may depend on who's doing the measuring. Dr. Dean Edell has a very interesting free newsletter at www.healthcentral.com. He recently had an article about penile sizes and measurements.

> "What's normal seems like a simple question. But when you look into the subject, you find that observations differ, depending on who's doing the measuring.

> "It should come as no surprise that a recent study from the University of California School of Medicine with the following data about penis sizes found that 'average' was considerably less than a group of men self-reporting their penile sizes on a Web site."

PHYSICIANS' FINDINGS

Physicians studied a group of 80 men to measure penis size when flaccid, stretched, and erect to establish guidelines for augmentation. The result? Only one man out of 80 was "even close" to the standard researchers defined as "subnormal."

Average Lengths
Flaccid—3.5 inch
Stretched—4.9 inch
Erect—5.1 inch

Average Circumference
Flaccid—3.9 inches
Erect—4.9 inches

Below Average
Erect Length—2.8 inches
Circumference 3.5 inches

INTERNET SELF-REPORTS FINDINGS

Meanwhile, data from an Internet site entitled "The Definitive Penis Size Survey, Sixth Edition" at http://www.connection.com/~dickie/result.html claims to have collected data from 3,100 site visitors. The site says its data is the "most exhaustive penis size survey to be conducted to date." The site's author says he has thrown out obvious cases of fraudulent responses such as respondents who claimed "American Zulu warrior" ancestry, for instance, from its reported results. They have a whole lot of data and charts at the site. One chart shows the percentage of men who are contented, or discontented with their size. About 75% of the below average or modestly endowed group were unhappy. About 20% of the average group were unhappy, and less than 10% of the well endowed group were unhappy.

There is an area at the site where you can send your measurements or make comments.

Here are some of the self-report findings at the web site.

Erect Length
Modest—5.6 inches
Average—6.4 inches
Endowed—7.1 inches

Erect Circumference
Modest—4.6 in
Average—5.0 in
Endowed—5.4 in

As you can see, the self-reported findings seem to find men who have penis sizes more than 1.5 inches longer than when physicians do the measuring!

Here are measuring guidelines that are used by physicians:

First, you need a tape measure. You'll want to measure the exact length of the penis from the meatus (that's the opening of the urethra) to the fat pad. The physicians from UCSF were careful to really push the fat pad down, and you should be, too. For the best results, take measurements of the penis in flaccid, stretched, and erect states. You'll get more reliable numbers.

Some inconsistencies will inevitably result. Flaccid measurements are less accurate than erect measurements. Cold or warm weather can also affect the findings.

Obesity can also affect the results. The team of UCSF researchers noted in their findings that, "The depth of the fat pad may significantly alter the perception of penile length. An increase in fat pad depth will decrease the visible pendulous length of the penis. Many men complain of a retractile penis, and obesity contributes to this phenomenon."

The researchers further stated that knowing the truth could reduce anxiety. "Knowledge of functional penile length," they wrote, "including that buried by the fat pad, may decrease anxiety concerning erect size in certain men."

They suggest that for men whose obesity is creating a perception of smaller penis size, weight loss or liposuction may represent less drastic steps to enhance a man's self-image about his penis size—i.e. fat is the real culprit.

Source: "Penile Length in the Flaccid and Erect States: Guidelines for Penile Augmentation," Journal of Urology, Vol. 195, 995-997, 1996.

It is so true that obesity and the fat pad around the base of the penis can rob you of some length.

I heard a story of two golfers who were taking a shower after the game. One of the men was very obese. The thin guy said, "Good God man, when is the last time you saw your penis? Why don't you diet?" The fat guy said, "Dye it? Hell, I don't even know what color it is now."

SURGICAL AUGMENTATION

It is not as easy for a man to have penile augmentation as it is for a woman to have her breasts enlarged. But there are several doctors who are doing it. The penis is one of the few organs or tissues of the body that has no fat. Several urologists are now performing a procedure for penile girth enlargement and a penile lengthening procedure.

For the girth enlargement procedure, they use a liposuction type technique to withdraw adipose, or fat cell tissue, from the man's abdomen, love handles or other fatty areas. This fat is then injected beneath the loose skin of the penis thus making it larger. The procedure requires no hospitalization. It can be done in the office in a fairly short time and is relatively painless.

They claim that they can enlarge the girth of the penis by 30 to 50 percent. Since the fat used is from the person's own body, there is no danger of rejection. But in most cases, the body will eventually absorb and remove the fat. However, the procedure can be repeated as often as the patient desires. Some urologists are using strips of skin with fat attached to enlarge the girth of the penis. It costs about $3500 for the girth enlargement procedure.

It is fairly easy to make the penis larger in girth but rather difficult to make it longer. For years, many companies of questionable repute have advertised in men's magazines with claims that they can lengthen the penis. They usually advertise a vacuum erection device similar to the device that I bought as an aid for my erections.

About one third of the penis is inside the body. It can be felt in the perineal area between the testicles and anus. In the front, the penis arches upward and is anchored to the pubic bone by suspensory ligaments. See fig. 4-1. On some men the penis can be lengthened up to one inch or more by cutting the suspensory ligaments.

Once the suspensory ligaments have been cut, the penis may flop from side to side and be rather unwieldy, but there will be more in front than before. There are several urologists in the Los Angeles area who have penile enlargement ads in the sport pages every day. Some of them also advertise in the *Penthouse* and other men's magazines. One doctor has been doing as many as 150 operations every month. Several of these doctors have become multi-millionaires.

But not every man has been satisfied with the treatments. Some have claimed to have a loss of feeling, lumpiness and ugly scarring in the penis. The California Medical Board has suspended the license of one doctor who was doing most of the procedures. But in defense of the doctors, there have been several thousand operations performed with only a few complaints.

This type of procedure is still fairly new and experimental. It will be some time before we know what the long-term effects will be.

Most men who have seen X-rated movies are bound to be a bit envious of the endowments of the men in those movies. But most men realize that the performers in those movies are not the average man. They were chosen because of their rare and exceptional endowments. However, it is possible to have too much of a good thing. I have seen photos of a man who has a penis that is 15 inches long. I am sure that he receives no more enjoyment from sex than any man with a small penis. Normal sex with this man would be very difficult for a woman.

A physically small body size does not necessarily mean that a man will have a small penis. Most short men have an average size penis. But Napoleon seemed to have been short-changed in both departments. When Napoleon died they cut off his penis and preserved it in a jar of alcohol. It was about two inches long. It is possible that because Napoleon was small in stature and penis size, that he compensated for it by trying to become the most powerful man on earth.

To most women size doesn't make that much difference. I am sure that Napoleon pleased Josephine. The vagina can conform to accommodate just about any size penis, or even to the passage of an eight pound baby. According to *Gray's Anatomy*, the length of the anterior wall of the vagina is 6 to 7.5 centimeters (cm) long and the length of the posterior wall is 9 cm long. One inch is equal to 2.54 centimeters, so if a woman is lying on her back, the upper wall of the vagina is 2.4 to 2.8 inches long and the rear wall is about 3.6 inches long.

This may seem strange, because very few men are able to ever "hit bottom." The reason is that the vagina is somewhat like the penis. During sexual arousal, the uterus is drawn upward and the vagina becomes longer and deeper. Masters and Johnson called it "tenting." So not only can it accommodate the girth of the largest penis, it can usually accommodate a very long penis.

Many women have found that by doing Kegel exercises they can strengthen the vaginal muscles so that they can squeeze down on even a very small penis.

Many men are ashamed of what they have. If you look at the men in a public rest room, most of them will go out of their way to try to hide it. They will practically climb into a urinal so the guy next to them won't be able to see. Many men even go into a stall and close the door so that no one can see them. But there are a few men who are showoffs. These are the ones who are well endowed and they want the whole world to know it. I once stood next to a very short and very homely man in a public rest room, but it seems that God must have compensated him in other ways. His endowment would have made a stud horse envious. The little guy shook it and flopped it around so that everyone in the rest room could see how lucky he was.

Successful reproduction does not depend on the length of the penis. If the only men who could father children were those with a long penis, then the male children would have inherited the genes for a long penis. Over the last few million years, evolution would have eliminated most of the men with short penises.

Most of the sensory nerves in the vagina are near the entrance. We mentioned the woman's "G" spot earlier. It is about one inch inside on the upper front part of the vagina. Stimulation of this area brings many women to orgasm. So most women only need about two or three inches for satisfaction. In fact many women don't even need penetration to have an orgasm. The clitoris is a rudimentary penis and can be stimulated much like a penis. Most women can have a stronger orgasm from oral and manual manipulation of the clitoris than from vaginal thrusting.

Of course there are some women who are turned on by a large penis and still think they need one. I heard a story once about a man who picked up a woman and took her to his room. When he got undressed, the woman laughed and said, "Who do you expect to make happy with that little thing?" The man replied, "Me."

So the length of the penis is not all that critical for enjoyment or for reproduction. Many women have become pregnant even when the sperm was deposited outside the vagina during a withdrawal method of birth control. When given a chance to find an egg, those little sperm are very determined.

There are some women who also may not be happy with their sex organs. I once visited the Steinhart aquarium in San Francisco with a lady friend. They had a large photo of a couple of whales in the act of mating. I said, "I have read that the lucky whale may have a penis as long as six feet." My lady friend said, "Yeah, well the unlucky female probably has a vagina that is ten feet deep." Such is life.

Chapter Five
BENIGN PROSTATIC HYPERPLASIA
Drs. Aubrey Pilgrim and E. David Crawford

Each year at the American Urological Association Convention, about 150 papers on BPH are presented. BPH is one of the most prevalent health problems among aging men. It has been estimated that about six million men in the United States over the age of 50 and another 17 million men world-wide suffer from BPH. The BPH symptoms include increased frequency of urination, a sudden urge to urinate and difficulty in urinating or a weak flow of urine. These symptoms may cause a diminished quality of life (QOL). It is possible that the excessive tissue growth can completely compress the urethra so that little or no urine can be passed. At this time, it definitely causes a diminished QOL.

In the United States, about a half million men each year are being treated for BPH with various types of surgery. More than 1.5 million men are being treated each year for BPH with drug therapy. To date, alpha-blockers have been considered the most effective pharmaceutical and non-surgical treatment for BPH. The single greatest cost to Medicare, at close to 3 billion dollars per year, is for cataract treatments. The next greatest cost, at over 2.5 billion dollars per year, is for BPH treatments. The greater expense for cataracts is because it includes both men and women and each of the two eyes are affected.

WHAT BPH IS
Benign prostatic hyperplasia (BPH) is a non-cancerous tumor. The prefix *hyper*—means above, beyond or excessive; the suffix—*plasia* means to form. Hyperplasia is defined as an abnormal increase in the volume of a tissue or organ caused by the formation and growth of normal cells. BPH is sometimes called benign prostatic hypertrophy. The suffix *trophy* means nourishment. So literally, hyper-

trophy would mean excessive nourishment. The term *benignus* or benign is Latin for mild. It is the opposite of *malignus* or malignant, which is Latin for bad. Even though BPH is not malignant, there are times when it can be rather bad if it prevents you from urinating.

The term urine is from the Latin *urina* and it is also related to the Greek *ouron*. Another term used often in the medical literature is *micturition*, which is from the Latin to pass urine. And of course common terms that mean the same thing are pee and piss which is usually considered a bit vulgar. (It seems strange to me that it's okay to say almost anything in Latin or Greek, such as coitus, feces, flatulence but the more common terms are vulgar.)

BPH is very common among older men. Four out of every five men between the ages of 50 and 60 will have enlargement of their prostate to some degree. It will be so enlarged in about 95 percent of the 80-year-old men that they may need treatment. It may grow so large that it constricts the prostatic urethra and obstructs the passage of urine. The constriction may be such that it causes urine to back up so that the kidneys cannot function properly.

RESIDUAL URINE

The obstruction may cause a pool of residual urine to remain in the bladder. This pool may stagnate and promote bacterial growth and lead to infections. If you can't entirely empty the bladder, you will feel as if you have to go, even though you have just urinated. The urologist may check for residual urine by having you drink a liquid that will show up on an X-ray. After drinking the liquid, you will be asked to wait until you have to urinate. Immediately after you urinate, they will take an X-ray of your bladder. If you have any residual urine, it will show on the X-ray.

The bladder is made up of muscles. If the patient has to constantly strain to force urine through the constricted urethra, it may cause the muscles in the bladder walls to thicken and become stronger. But even the stronger bladder muscles may not be able to completely empty the bladder so that a pool of residual urine is left. In some cases as much as three or four ounces is retained in the bladder after voiding. Bacterial infections may arise from the residual pool and may cause the formation of bladder stones.

We are all different. In some cases the prostate may severely constrict the urethra even though it is not enlarged to any great degree. In other cases the prostate may be quite enlarged, yet cause no trouble.

CATHETERIZATION

BPH is a condition that has always affected older men. Over four thousand years ago the Egyptians used a hollow reed from those that grew along the Nile river as a catheter for men who had BPH. As any man might imagine, shoving a reed into the penile urethra is not very pleasurable. If you look at the drawing of fig. 4-1, you will see that the urethra is not a straight path. If the penis is held out straight, the path of the urethra curves downward and then upward through the prostate. Today we have flexible catheters. Of course they had no anesthetics in those days, so the men would wait as long as possible before submitting to the painful procedure. Usually several men had to hold the man down while the reed was inserted. The reed catheter would not cure the BPH, but it would give the patient a short spell of relief until his bladder filled again.

If the urethral obstruction becomes so great that no urine passes through, it then becomes a life-threatening emergency. This is what killed Thomas Jefferson and several other men years ago. We now have several treatments that are much better and less painful than the Nile reed. If the patient cannot pass urine, he can be hospitalized and catheterized with a flexible tube. The normal bladder may hold about one pint. The bladder is highly distensible, but can be very painful when the normal limits are exceeded. There have been cases where as much as four quarts of urine have been drained from a catheterized man. It makes me shudder just to think about this.

BPH VS PROSTATE CANCER

BPH is merely a proliferation of normal prostate cells. In the vast majority of men over 50 years old, the whole prostate begins to enlarge. In prostate cancer, a tumor of abnormal cells begin to form. At first it is a small tumor, but it may eventually grow so large that it infiltrates and occupies the entire prostate. A large cancer growth may also cause the urethra to be constricted and blocked to the same extent as BPH.

Another difference is that the BPH tumor may still be fairly soft and pliable. A cancer tumor may be made up of very tightly packed cells. During a digital rectal exam, (DRE), when the doctor puts his gloved finger in the rectum, he can usually detect the difference in the soft normal tissue or BPH and the hard lumpy cancer tissue.

Unlike the normal BPH cells, the cancer cells are not normal functioning cells. Another difference is that the prostate cancer has the capability of infiltrating nearby tissues and organs and metastasizing to distant sites. BPH stays within the prostate capsule but it sometimes grows so large that it pushes up and presses on the bladder. This pressure and squeezing can partially collapse the bladder and will decrease the volume of urine that the bladder can store. It may also cause a pool to be formed so that some residual urine is retained after the patient has voided.

BPH is much more common than prostate cancer. About 500,000 men will be newly diagnosed with BPH this year. This is in addition to the 1.5 million who are being treated from having been diagnosed in previous years. About 180,000 men will be diagnosed with prostate cancer this year. Another 3 million will have prostate cancer, but may not be aware of it or have any symptoms.

BPH GROWTH

The prostate has a tough fibrous capsule that surrounds it. As the BPH cells proliferate, they soon fill all of the space within the capsule. As they continue to multiply, they are somewhat limited in their outward growth by the prostatic capsule. The cells continue to multiply so they constrict the urethra that passes through the middle of the prostate. There may be several degrees of constriction. BPH can make it difficult to pee. In some cases it will only cause a diminished flow of urine. In other cases the urethra may be so constricted that the man can only pass urine with great difficulty or not at all. You have probably seen concrete sidewalks that have been buckled up and broken by the growth of tree roots. The increase in the number of cells in a tree's roots can exert enough pressure to break a four-inch thick concrete sidewalk. The cells in your body are basically quite similar to the cells in a tree root. So you can understand how the prostate cells can overcome the constraints of the prostatic capsule. The prostate may grow from the size of a chestnut, or about ¾ ounce to the size of a large orange. Dr. August Roumani says that he removed an enlarged prostate that weighed over 600 grams. (One ounce is 28.35 grams, one pound is 454 grams so this prostate weighed approximately 1¼ pounds.)

PROSTATE DEVELOPMENT

Most glands in the body grow to a certain size then stop growing. The prostate is about the size of a pea at birth, but it continues to grow and become larger throughout a man's life. Early growth was due to testosterone but as a man ages, there is less testosterone. Since there is less testosterone, there must be some other factor that causes the increased growth of BPH and prostate cancer in older men.

The prostate cells cannot utilize testosterone until it has been converted to dihydrotestosterone (DHT). An enzyme, 5 alpha-reductase, metabolizes the testosterone and converts it to DHT. Some males are born without the ability to produce the 5 alpha-reductase enzyme. The testosterone that they produce cannot be converted to DHT so they never have BPH or prostate cancer. Proscar is a 5 alpha-reductase inhibitor. It is widely used as a treatment for BPH.

Testosterone is also a factor in baldness. A young man who has been castrated will never go bald or have prostate cancer. Merck, the company who makes the Proscar drug, also makes Propecia, a drug used for baldness treatments. Propecia is the same as Proscar but in a smaller dosage.

There are certain specific receptors in the prostate that combine with the DHT. During the normal aging process, the number of receptors should decline, along with the decline of testosterone and other body functions. But it appears that these receptors are not affected by aging. Even though there is a decline in testosterone, there may be even more receptors available for using a greater percentage of the testosterone that is present. This could explain why the prostate continues to grow throughout life.

There is a similar problem with breast cancer in women. It proliferates in the presence of the female hormone estrogen. Yet it is most prevalent in women over 50 years of age who have gone through menopause and have stopped producing estrogen. There is a whole lot about the human body and cancer that we still don't know. It may be that there are similar specific receptors in women that promotes breast cancer.

SYMPTOMS AND SIGNS OF BPH

Here are some of the symptoms of BPH. Depending on your age, you may have some or all of these symptoms, but you may not need treatment. Most of the following symptoms may also be present in prostate cancer.

Diuria—The need to urinate frequently during the day

Normally you shouldn't have to go more than once every two hours during the day unless you drink a lot of liquids such as coffee, tea or beer. The prostate may be so large that it is pressing on the bladder so that it's capacity is diminished. The normal bladder in a man should have a capacity of 12 to 17 ounces. (Most medical measurements are listed in milliliters (ml) or cubic centimeters (cc) which are both the same. One oz. is 29.57 ml or 29.57 cc. The normal bladder will hold from 355 ml or cc and up to 502 ml or cc.)

Nocturia—Getting up two or more times at night

Most men, and a lot of women, have to get up at least once during the night, especially if they have had a lot to drink in the evening before bed time. But men who have BPH may have to get up several times during the night. He may only void a small amount each time. It is possible that the prostate has become so enlarged that it presses on the bladder and prevents it from holding as much as it normally should. Nocturia is the most common BPH symptom that causes men to see their doctor.

Nocturia is not a guarantee that you do or do not have BPH. Even if a person has had a radical prostatectomy, he still may have to get up two or more times at night.

Urgency, feeling that you cannot wait

You may have the feeling that you cannot wait. It may feel as if your bladder will burst before you can get to the toilet.

Hesitancy or Difficulty in starting the urine

If you have to stand there for more than five or six seconds trying to find the right button to push, it could be a sign that all is not well below. Of course, the time and place may also make a difference. If you are in a crowded public restroom and you think everyone is staring at you and your equipment, finding the right button to push may be difficult even if you don't have BPH.

Straining

You may have to strain to force urine through the constricted urethra. This can cause thickened bladder muscles. Constant straining may also cause the bladder muscles to simply give up and not work at all.

Many men wake up in the morning with an erection and an urge to urinate (a pee hard on). In this case you almost always have to strain to get it started. The reason is that the bladder sphincter, or valve, is supposed to remain closed in the presence of an erection. This is to prevent any ejaculate that might occur from entering the bladder. After a transurethral resection prostatectomy (TURP) this valve is usually damaged. In this case, quite often when an ejaculation occurs, the semen takes the shorter route into the bladder. This is called retrograde emission. We will discuss it in more detail later.

Dribbling and difficulty in stopping

It is bad enough that you may have trouble starting it, but you may not be able to stop it. At least, not completely. A person with BPH may think that he is all finished. He may stand there and shake it for five minutes, but the minute he puts it away and zips up, it will leak all over the front of his pants. If you are late for an important meeting or in a hurry, it will be even worse than usual. It can be terribly embarrassing.

Decreased size or caliber of the stream

A young man may have a stream that seems to be about a fourth of an inch in diameter. A man who has BPH may have a stream less than a sixteenth of an inch in diameter. This would be due to the constriction of the prostatic portion of the urethral tube.

Decreased strength and force of the stream

When I was young I could stand at one end of an open trough type public urinal and knock a fly off the wall ten feet away. My stream was so weak before my prostatectomy that I couldn't disturb a fly that was as close as one foot away.

Feeling as though you still have to go

You may have just finished, but you may still feel like you have to go.

Dysuria—Pain or burning during urination

Any pain or burning sensation could be due to irritation of the urethra. If the patient is unable to completely empty the bladder, it may lead to bacterial infection which may cause pain and burning during urination. Pain and burning could also indicate that you have an inflammation, prostatitis, bladder stones or prostatic stones.

Squat to pee

When I was young, calling a boy a sissy was about the worst thing you could call him. When we really wanted to put a guy down we would say that he was such a sissy that he had to squat to pee. If you have difficulty in peeing, you might try to do it squatting or sitting on the commode. In some men it seems to help relieve the obstruction a bit. Just be sure to close the bathroom door so that nobody will see you and call you a sissy.

Complete retention of urine

This is an emergency situation. The patient should be immediately hospitalized and treated.

Nausea, dizziness, unusual sleepiness

These symptoms may occur if there has been kidney damage due to the urine blockage.

Tabulating Your Symptoms

You can do a self evaluation. Rate the symptoms in Table 5.1 from 0 to 5 as to how you are affected by each one. If you rated each of the 7 items at the maximum 5, you could have a score of 35. If you come any where close to this number, you should definitely see your doctor. Of course, you don't really need a score card to know whether you have a problem or not.

This table is now used worldwide. It is sometimes referred to as IPSS for International Prostate Symptom Score. (The IPSS acronym is almost dirty, but seems rather apropos.)

TABLE 5-1

AUA INTERNATIONAL PROSTATE SYMPTOM SCORE INDEX

Question During Last Month	Not at All	Less Than 1 Time in 5	Less Than Half The Time	About Half The Time	More than Half The Time	Almost Always
1. How often have you had a sensation of not emptying your bladder completely after you finished urinating.	0	1	2	3	4	5
2. Had to urinate again within 2 hours	0	1	2	3	4	5
3. Had to stop and start several times	0	1	2	3	4	5
4. Was difficult to hold it—had to go now	0	1	2	3	4	5
5. Had a weak urinary stream	0	1	2	3	4	5
6. Had to strain to urinate	0	1	2	3	4	5
7. Number of times got up at night	0	1	2	3	4	5

BPH DIAGNOSIS

There are several tests that the doctor will perform to determine whether you have BPH.

DRE

One of the most common tests that a doctor does is the digital rectal exam (DRE). The examination may be a bit embarrassing, but it is quick and easy and can yield an enormous amount of information. The patient bends over on the examining table and the doctor inserts a lubricated gloved finger into the rectum. The posterior and lateral lobes of the prostate can be easily felt through the thin rectal wall. The normal prostate should be about the size of a chestnut and should feel smooth and elastic. The doctor can determine if the size of the prostate is larger than normal. Even though it is larger than normal, it should still feel smooth and elastic if the enlargement is caused by BPH. If the doctor finds any hard nodules or areas of undue firmness, then he may suspect cancer.

A doctor may not be able to positively determine if a patient has BPH by DRE alone. The doctor can only feel the two rear lobes of the prostate.

The middle lobe, which lies in the front portion of the prostate, could be obstructive, but it cannot be felt. Unfortunately, the front middle lobe is the most common site for obstructions that cause BPH symptoms.

Flow Rate Test

If the urethra becomes constricted because of BPH it will cause a reduction in the amount of urine that can be voided in a given amount of time. The stream may gradually become very small and the man may not be aware of it. An important test is to check the flow rate.

The doctor may have you undergo a uroflowmetry test. You will be asked to drink a large amount of water. When you can't hold it any longer the doctor will have you void into a measured container. The container may be part of a very complex computerized test instrument. The instrument can calculate the instant the first drop hits the bottom, then calculates the time until you stop. The uroflowmeter measures the volume of urine that is voided and the amount of time that it takes per milliliter (ml). They usually need about 200 ml to have a valid test. (200 ml is about 7 ounces.) A normal man under 40 years old should be able to fill a 7 ounce cup in about nine seconds, or about 22 ml/second. A normal man between 40 and 60 should be able to fill it in about 11 seconds or about 18 ml/second. A normal man over 60 will need a little over 15 seconds or about 13 ml/second. A man who has BPH may need 20 to 40 seconds to pass 200 ml, depending on the severity of the urethral constriction.

The computerized uroflowmeter or urodynamic system may be rather expensive. At the AUA 2000 Convention, one company had a very expensive urodynamic system. It had a chair similar to a dentist chair, except that it had a v shaped slot in the front. Under this slot was a large funnel and bucket. There was a flouroscope system that focused on the pelvic area and all of this was connected to a computer. The whole system was priced at a mere $180,000.

The whole idea of the urodynamic system is to determine how fast a man can void a given amount. But one can do about the same thing by using a 7 ounce cup and a stop watch. Just drink a lot of water, then use the watch to see how long it takes to fill a cup. Many doctors may use a simple stop watch or a watch with a second hand and a glass beaker with graduated markings. Many people have a shy bladder and have difficult in starting it if someone is watching or timing them. You may be given a stopwatch and asked to time yourself in a private lavatory, which is a whole lot less expensive than the $180,000 system.

It is important that these urodynamic tests be performed before any treatment is begun. Once the doctor has an idea of the scope of your problem, he may begin a series of treatments. Every so often the urodynamic tests can be repeated and checked against the original test to determine if the treatment is having any effect. If there is no change in the rate of urine flow, then the doctor may change the treatments.

DO YOUR OWN HOME TESTS

You can do your own tests at home by using a measuring cup and a watch with a second hand. Drink a lot of water, then wait as long as you can to go. Most measuring cups, such as the glass Pyrex cups, have markings in both ounces and in milliliters. It is not necessary to be absolutely precise in these measurements. Your wife may get pissed off if you pee in one of her good measuring cups so you could use something such as a styrofoam or paper cup. Just measure out 7 ounces of water and mark the cup. If you have BPH it will be obvious.

POST VOID RESIDUAL (PVR) URINE

As the obstruction of the prostatic urethra becomes greater, the patient may not be able to completely empty his bladder. He may be able to start to void, but his small stream may stop for a few seconds and then it may start again. This often happens when the man thinks he is finished, shakes it a few times, then puts it away. But the minute he zips up, urine will run down his leg and wet his pants. He may stand there and strain but he still may have residual urine left in the bladder even after it wets his clothes.

There are several ways to detect residual urine. When your doctor examines you, he may feel your lower abdomen to determine if there is residual urine in your bladder. The doctor may have you void as much as you can and then he may use a catheter or a cystoscope to drain the residual urine and measure it. In severe cases, there may be as much as a pint or even a quart of post void residual (PVR) urine.

The doctor may order an x-ray urogram. The patient is usually injected with a contrast dye that will show up on an x-ray. Several x-rays may be taken as the dye-colored liquid is filtered out of the blood and collected in the bladder. Finally, the patient is asked to void, and then another x-ray is taken which can show any urine left in the bladder.

ULTRASONIC IMAGING

Your doctor may also use an ultrasound machine to determine residual urine. A residual pool of urine can be seen on the ultrasound image. The ultrasound can be used to view the enlarged prostate. Cancerous tumor images can also be seen with ultrasound.

MRI AND CT

Magnetic resonance imaging (MRI) machines or computed tomography (CT) machines can also be used. But these machines are very expensive and would probably only be used if there were difficulties in the diagnosis or other complications.

CYSTOSCOPIC EXAMINATION

Your doctor may also want to do a cystoscopic examination. The prefix cyst is from the Greek *kystis* which means bladder or sac. The cystoscope is a tubular instrument that can be used to examine the interior of the bladder and other body cavities. It has thin fiber optics which can conduct light and a magnifying lens at the end. The doctor can insert this instrument into the urethra and examine any obstruction in the prostate. He can also examine the interior of the bladder for residual urine, for muscle irregularities and for bladder stones. There are several different types of the cystoscope. It may be fitted with grasping forceps or with a cutting scalpel. The cystoscope has an eyepiece that the doctor can look through, but it may also have provisions to electronically display the image on a television screen.

There are also several different diameters for cystoscopes, catheters, probes and sounds which are measured by the French scale. This scale was devised by a Frenchman named Chevrrier. The English people had trouble pronouncing and spelling his name so the scale came to be known simply as the French scale. Each unit is about 1/3 millimeter so that a 21 French, or 21F, cystoscope is 7 mm in diameter. One mm is .04 inches so 7 mm would be .28 inches or a little more than a quarter of an inch in diameter. It wouldn't be too difficult to insert a 21F cystoscope into the urethra. But many cystoscopes and probes may be a half inch or more in diameter. It makes me shudder to even think of something a half inch in diameter being inserted in my urethra. Fortunately, the doctors may use anesthesia with these instruments.

PSA

The doctor may order a urine test and a blood test to rule out any infection. The blood sample may also be tested for the presence of prostatic specific antigen (PSA). The normal prostate may produce PSA from .2 nanograms per milliliter (ng/ml) of blood and up to 4.0 ng/ml. An enlarged prostate due to BPH may produce as much as 10 ng/ml or more. A cancerous prostate tumor that is the same size and mass as a BPH tumor will usually produce about ten times more PSA than the BPH tumor.

More about PSA in the next chapter.

BIOPSY

The doctor may want to do a biopsy to make sure that the enlarged prostate is benign. He may use a spring loaded needle through the wall of the rectum to retrieve a sample of the prostate cells. He may take several samples from different areas of the prostate. It is fairly painless. The samples are sent to a pathology lab for microscopic inspection.

TREATMENTS FOR BPH

There are several different treatments for BPH. Many treatments involve surgery, but there are also several treatments using devices that are non-surgical. There are also several drugs that are used. Each type of treatment has its advantages and usually some disadvantages.

SURGICAL TREATMENTS

Surgical treatments may include suprapubic and retropubic prostatectomies. A simple prostatectomy and a radical prostatectomy are very much different procedures. The suffix—*ectomy* means excision of an organ or gland, but not necessarily the complete organ or gland. A radical prostatectomy means the complete excision and removal of the gland. A radical prostatectomy or complete removal of the prostate, is seldom done for treatment of BPH.

TURP

Radical prostatectomy has been called the "Gold Standard" for prostate cancer. The Transurethral Resection Prostate (TURP) has been called the "Platinum Standard" for BPH. It uses a resectoscope which utilizes a wire loop and electrocautery to remove tissue. Several crude instruments were made as early as 1888. Many improvements were made by several different men over the next 44 years. In 1932 a man named McCarthy took the best of all the earlier developments and introduced a resectoscope that is basically the same instrument used today. Of course newer lenses and fiberoptics have been added.

The resectoscope is a tube that is about 12 inches long and about a half inch in diameter. The tube contains wires for the electrocautery loop, a light source, and a tube for irrigating water. The normal urethra is about one fourth of an inch in diameter. The patient must be anesthetized in order to force the half inch resectoscope into the urethra. The surgeon looks through the eyepiece and can see the obstructive portions of the prostatic urethra. He uses the wire loop to snip off pieces of the obstruction. Water is used to flush the cut pieces into the bladder. The electric wire loop cauterizes the tissue so that there is little or no bleeding.

The operation may require about an hour and a half. After the operation, the cut pieces of tissue are flushed out of the bladder and sent to a pathology laboratory to be examined for cancer cells. Cancer is found in about 10% of all cases. In many cases, the cancer is a type that seems to be non aggressive. Often, no treatment is necessary except to watch and wait. The patient's PSA can be monitored, and if it rises, then appropriate action may be taken. If the cells appear to be an aggressive type of cancer, the urologist may recommend that the patient have a radical prostatectomy.

After the operation a Foley catheter is inserted through the urethra and into the bladder. The Foley catheter has a small balloon on the bladder end that is filled with water to hold it in place. The catheter is left in place several days to give the prostate a chance to heal.

A TURP usually requires one or more days of hospitalization which can add to the overall cost of the procedure.

ADVERSE SIDE EFFECTS

Bleeding And Infection

There may be some bleeding, and it is possible that the patient may need at least one unit of transfused blood. With the AIDS fears of today, the doctor may suggest that the patient make an autologous donation of his own blood. If the patient needs it, his own blood would be much better for him.

There is also a chance of infection during the operation. Fortunately, most infections can be controlled by penicillin and other drugs.

Incontinence

All patients will have incontinence to some degree after a TURP. Most patients will overcome it a short time. The reason for the incontinence is that the prostate is closely tied to the bladder. The bladder sphincter is usually damaged to some degree. If the surgeon is not very careful, it may be damaged severely.

Retrograde Ejaculation

Ordinarily during sexual arousal, the bladder sphincter is tightly closed. But if the bladder sphincter has been damaged, it may not be able to close. In this case, during ejaculation, the semen and sperm take the much shorter route into the bladder. The man will have the same orgasmic sensation as before, but the ejaculate ends up in the bladder.

TUIP

A transurethral incision prostatectomy (TUIP) is a fairly simple procedure where cuts or slits are made in the prostatic portion of the urethra. This operation may be less traumatic than a TURP and have less side effects, but it may not be effective in all cases.

The slits are usually made with a special scalpel, but they may also be done with a laser.

The word laser is an acronym for Light Amplification by Stimulated Emission of Radiation. Ordinary light is made up of random incoherent wave lengths. A laser beam is made up of a single amplified coherent wave length. There are several different types of lasers. Some are powerful enough to burn a hole through a diamond. Several types have been adapted for surgical procedures. There are several advantages to laser surgery. One advantage is that the laser coagulates and seals blood vessels so that there is little or no bleeding. The strength of the laser is dependent on the amount of electrical power fed to it. By controlling the input power, the depth of a cut or ablation can be monitored and controlled.

TUMT

Transurethral microwave thermotherapy (TUMT) seems to be a good alternative to surgery. If the prostate cells are subjected to temperatures of about 45 degrees C or 113 degrees F, they will die. The source of the hyperthermia is high frequency microwaves similar to those used in home microwave cooking ovens. But don't consider crawling into a microwave oven to cure your BPH. (On a recent Jay Leno show, Jay mentioned that microwaves are now being used to treat prostate problems. His sidekick, Kevin the band leader, asked, "How does one get his ass in a microwave?")

The microwave instrument systems are designed so that the temperature and the depth of heating are exactly controlled. A report presented at the 1993 AUA convention listed results of 150 patients who had been treated with TUMT. The patients were subjected to a 45 degree C temperature for about 60 minutes. There was no need for anesthesia, or hospitalization. There was little or no bleeding and little pain. There were no reports of retrograde ejaculation or significant changes in sexual function. The procedure has been used in foreign countries for some time and has just recently been approved by the FDA for use in the US. It would seem possible that TUMT could be used for types of prostate cancer.

It appears to offer very good results. The procedure offers an alternative for those men who are not good candidates for surgery.

TUNA

No, it is not the fish. It means Transurethral Needle Ablation. It uses a low level radio frequency (RF) of about 490kHz to create a temperature of 50 to 90 degrees C in the area to be ablated. The probe is a special catheter which has two flexible needles at the tip. The needles can be deployed and inserted into the prostate through the urethra. The needles are about 45 degrees apart. They are shielded at their base so that the urethral tissue is not damaged. When the RF energy is turned on, it passes from one needle to the other so that the prostatic tissue between the needles is destroyed. The progress of the treatment can be viewed on a TRUS. The needles can be repositioned so that many areas of the prostate can be treated. The treatment can be an outpatient procedure with local anesthesia. The patient can leave soon after the treatment.

DRUG TREATMENTS

Testosterone and BPH

Testosterone is both a blessing and a bane. It is the hormone that makes us horny and hunger for sex. Even women must have a bit of testosterone to have a desire for sex. Without this hormone, not many of us would be here. But prostate cancer and the excessive growth of cells in BPH is directly related to the male hormone testosterone. The prostate cells proliferate and may grow in excessive numbers in the presence of this hormone. If the source of testosterone is removed, many of the prostate cells will wither and die. Of course the source of testosterone is the testes. A man who has been castrated in early life will never have BPH or prostate cancer. Many of the treatments for BPH and prostate cancer are designed to eliminate, hinder or counteract the action of the male hormones.

Hytrin, Minipress, Flomax and Cardura

There are several high blood pressure drugs, called alpha blockers, that act on the nervous system to relax the arteries. Quite often patients with BPH also present with hypertension or high blood pressure. These drugs also have an effect on the smooth muscle of the prostate to some extent. Some of the blood pressure drugs used to treat BPH are Hytrin, Minipress and Cardura.

The prostate is a musculo-glandular organ. It is interlaced with smooth muscle, much like the tubular musculature of the arteries. The smooth muscles of the arteries are controlled by the body's nervous system. One disadvantage of the alpha blockers is that they may not be effective on some prostates. Another disadvantage is that many of the alpha blockers may cause impotence problems.

A Little Booze for BPH

A study using ethanol alcohol for BPH was presented at the 1999 AUA meeting. Ethyl or ethanol alcohol is the drinking kind, it is normally about 80 proof or 40 percent ethanol. The ethanol used for this procedure was absolute or 200 proof. (It probably makes no difference whether it is scotch or bourbon). Methyl alcohol is usually distilled from wood. One should never drink methyl alcohol. It can make one go blind. The ethanol was injected into the prostate and it caused the tissues to atrophy and die.

Unproven and Untested Drugs

We are now in the age of alternative drugs, herbs and medicines. There is no question that there are some very good herbs and alternative medicines that have some merit. But there seems to be a large segment of the population that believes that many herbs and drugs have almost magical powers to cure everything. Most of the drugs and herbs that are for sale at the local health food store have never been properly studied and evaluated. Many people swear that some of these alternative medicines have benefited them greatly. It is possible that some of the benefits that these people receive are due to a placebo effect. Some studies indicate that any kind of drug or sugar pill will have a good or placebo effect about 40% of the time.

If you want to take the alternative drugs and herbs, please check with your doctor first. Some of them may cause an interaction with your conventional drugs. Most of these drugs probably won't harm you, but most of them won't do you much good either.

Here are some of the drugs and herbs that are supposed to help BPH.

Saw Palmetto

The Saw Palmetto Berry is supposed to do the same thing naturally that the Proscar drug does. No definitive scientific studies have been done in the US. Some studies were supposedly done in France in the early 1970s. Saw Palmetto is usually sold in health food stores. Since it is not FDA approved or controlled, there is no guarantee of the USP standards for purity or potency.

Essiac Tea

Essiac Tea has been around for some time. A woman named Caisse first made it from roots and herbs. It is supposed to cure BPH, prostate cancer and just about everything else. Essiac is Caisse spelled backwards.

Prostata

Prostata is a vitamin and mineral formulation that contains the saw palmetto berry, zinc and several other herbs and natural drugs. The company that manufactures prostata goes to great lengths to procure mailing lists of those men who have BPH or prostate cancer. They then mail out slick brochures with lots of testimonials from "satisfied users." The ads claim that the drug will prevent prostate cancer and alleviate the effects of BPH. No scientific studies have been done to corroborate any of their claims. They rely on their glowing testimonials instead. I am leery of any ad that has lots of testimonials.

There are many other alternative medicines on the market. If you must try them, use caution. By all means continue to take any medicines that have been prescribed for you.

Here are some alternative treatments for BPH from a web site written by Emily Kane, ND (Dr. of Naturopathy). She also has treatments for prostatitis, prostate cancer and several other diseases. Here is the URL for her site: http://www.naturopathic.org/articles.lay/EK.prostate.html

COLOR THERAPY

Color therapy is used most often with thin pieces of colored plastic ("gels") over home or office light sources, such as a lamp. The following colors are listed for BPH:

lemon (helps to dissolve blood clots; acts as a chronic alternative) on front of body; orange (acts as a decongestant) and indigo (an astringent, antipyic, antiemetic, and hemostatic) between genital and anal areas; indigo and violet on prostate; alternate blue and yellow on kidneys for 10 minutes each; drink blue treated water; violet on chest

STONES

A growing number of progressive thinkers like to use semiprecious stones for their healing. The stones may be held, or placed on the affected body part, or placed into the bottom of your drinking water. Consult someone who knows about "healing rocks" for more ideas. Here are a few used in BPH:

Coral, Pearl, Diamond, Topaz , Carnelian, Citrine, Ruby, Garnet

PSYCHOSPIRITUAL

The mind is by far the most important aspect in your total well-being. Psychospiritual approaches to healthcare are being used increasingly even in the most conventional of settings. The following ideas about the origins and treatment of BPH should provide some food for thought:

Sexual disturbances associated with chronic masturbation, prior STDs, extramarital affairs with unexpressed guilt feelings and long standing unhappy relationships; Unhappiness; Prostate represents masculine principle; Mental fears weaken the masculinity; Giving up; Sexual pressure and guilt; Belief in aging; Visualization.

Closing thoughts: What is the symptom preventing me from doing? What is the symptom making me do?

There is a whole lot more of this sort of thing on her site. There are dozens of other sites that offer similar alternative treatments for BPH, all kinds of cancer and any other disease known and unknown to man. To find other sites, just use any of the search engines such as www.excite.com, www.lycos.com, www.yahoo.com, www.altavista.com or any of the other search engines and search for BPH and Alternative medicine.

From what I have seen of the alternative medicines, the people who benefit most are those who sell them.

DRUG VS. SURGERY COSTS

At one of the American Urological Association (AUA) conventions,Dr. Terrence Malloy compared surgical methods to drugs for BPH treatment. In the short term, drugs appear to have a cost benefit over surgery. But the drugs may have to be continued for a long period of time. Here are some drug costs and other treatmentsthat he gave for the Philadelphia area:

Drugs

	Dosage	Per Month	Per Year
Proscar	5 mg	$75	$900
Hytrin	5 mg	$60	$720
Cardura	2 mg	$40	$480
Flomax	.4 mg	$50	$600

You should be aware that sometimes other drugs are prescribed in combination with Proscar, for instance Proscar and Hytrin. In this case, the cost for one year would be $1620.

Surgical Costs

Cost for a TUIP usually requires an overnight stay at a hospital, a TURP may require at least one day or more in the hospital. Of course this adds to the overall cost of the procedures.

The cost of TUNA and several other laser ablation treatments may be done as office procedures so the hospital costs could be avoided.

The cost of the office procedures may vary considerably depending on the surgeon. They may range from $6000 up to $15,000 or more. These operations may take less than an hour, but the electronic instruments needed for these procedures may be very expensive. And the doctor must include cost of nurses, receptionists, office space and other overhead costs.

The cost for a TURP is more expensive because the hospital costs must be included. A TURP may cost from $15,000 up to $20,000 or more.

The big advantage of surgery over drugs is that the surgery usually cures the BPH and is therefore a one-time cost. About 10% of the surgery patients will have to undergo an additional procedure.

Sometimes there is scarring and strictures due to surgery that requires additional treatment. Often this can be relieved by simply stretching the area with a balloon like device.

WATCHFUL WAITING

Depending on the severity of your BPH, you may not want to do anything. Almost every treatment has some side effects. And they all cost money and time. You must decide whether to suffer the consequences and side effects of treatment or whether you can live with the bother of your BPH.

Alas, life is full of compromises.

CHRONIC PROSTATITIS

Prostatitis affects a large number of men. In some cases, it may be very difficult to clear up. Many cases do respond to antibiotics.

IT PAYS TO ADVERTISE

Here are a couple of personalized license plates spotted in California:

CME2PEE...See Me To Pee, seen by Jerry Bostick

FNOPCME...If No P C Me, seen by Greg Holmes

Chapter Six

DIAGNOSIS AND STAGING

Drs. E. David Crawford and Aubrey Pilgrim

You may have arrived at the urologist's office because of several different events. Your general practitioner doc may have felt something a bit out of the ordinary when he or she did a digital rectal exam (DRE) for the annual checkup. You may have come because you participated in one of the screening efforts such as those promoted by the Prostate Cancer Awareness Week (PCAW). Or you may have come because you were having some bone pain. We sincerely hope that it was not for the latter reason.

SYMPTOMS

One reason so many men die from prostate cancer is that there may be no symptoms at all, or they may be very minor. Quite often the man may ignore the minor symptoms as just a part of the process of growing old. This could be a mistake that could cost years of his life. Often, by the time there are any symptoms, the cancer has already escaped the prostate gland and metastasized. That is why it is necessary to have regular checkups, even though you may feel fine. We have said it several times before, if it is found in time, it can be cured. **The Answer to Cancer is Early Detection.**

Many of the signs and symptoms of prostate cancer are the same as those listed for BPH in Chapter Five. You may have some or all of these symptoms without having prostate cancer. If you did not read that chapter, please turn back and read about the symptoms. Here is a brief list of them:

Diuria—The need to urinate frequently during the day

Nocturia—Getting up two or more times at night

Urgency, feeling that you cannot wait

Hesitancy or difficulty in starting the urine
Straining dribbling and difficulty in stopping
Decreased size or caliber of the stream
Decreased strength and force of the stream
Feeling as though you still have to go
Dysuria—Pain or burning during urination

If you have two or more of these symptoms, and if you haven't had a checkup recently, you should see your urologist.

DIAGNOSTIC TOOLS

No matter what brought you to the urologist, he or she will try to determine whether you actually have prostate cancer and, if you do, what is the stage. Doctors have several diagnostic tools to help in the diagnosis and staging of prostate cancer. Some prostate cancers may be rather difficult to detect. Separately, none of the tests are 100 percent accurate.

Prostate cancer cells go through several stages of development somewhat similar to the progression from being a baby to an old man. The cancer may start out as a single cell with a slight mutation. As it reproduces, the mutation becomes more and more pronounced as shown by Dr. Gleason's chart as it goes from grade 1 to 5. See fig. 6-1.

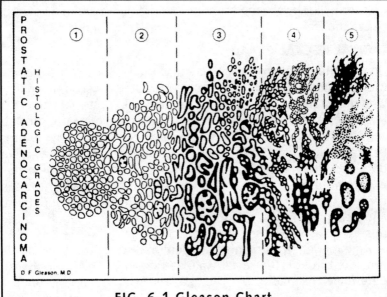

FIG. 6-1 Gleason Chart

Once the cancer is discovered, the doctor will perform several tests to gather as much information as possible. Once all the information is gathered, a clinical stage (CS) will be assigned such as T2b or B1. The stage describes the cancer and helps to make a decision as to what might be the best treatment.

The clinical stage (CS) of the cancer is only an estimate of the stage of the disease based on the tests, observations and best information available to the physician. It is not possible to determine absolutely what the clinical stage might be without removing the prostate and examining it under a microscope. If the prostate has been removed, a pathologist will examine it and assign a pathological stage, which would be indicated by a small p such as pT2b. In many cases, the clinical stage and pathological stage will be different. The man may be under staged or over staged clinically.

When you see your doctor, one of the first things that will probably be done, after you have filled out all the endless forms and paperwork, is to have blood drawn for a prostate specific antigen (PSA) test. The doctor may also ask that a prostate acid phosphatase (PAP) test be done from the same blood draw. This test was the first blood test used to detect prostate cancer and follow the course of the disease. Unfortunately it is not utilized that much anymore. It does supply some important information in some patients. Doctors may do a DRE first, then draw blood. Some believe that any rough manipulation or palpation of the prostate may cause a rise in the PSA. We have studied the effect of a routine screening exam on serum PSA levels and found that it did not result in a spurious rise in the PSA.

DIGITAL RECTAL EXAM

Up until the middle of the 1980s, the digital rectal exam (DRE) was the most common way to diagnose prostate cancer. In those days when prostate cancer was first diagnosed, in up to 70 percent of the patients the cancer had already metastasized. Early prostate cancer usually does not cause any pain or have any symptoms. Before we had the PSA test and more publicity, many men never bothered to have checkups until it got to the point where they experienced pain due to the cancer. At that time, usually the cancer had already metastasized. Even today despite lots of publicity and health warnings, many men still do not have regular checkups.

An experienced urologist can determine a lot from feeling the prostate through the rectal wall. See fig. 6-2. The urologist can determine the size of the prostate and if there are any unusual bumps or nodules. In his book, *Prostate Disease*, Dr. W. Scott McDougal says that the prostate should feel…"smooth, firm and a bit rubbery to the touch, much like the tip of the nose. So physicians let their fingers look for any irregularities like a bump or hard patch on the prostate. Not finding one is a good sign, but it's no guarantee that the gland is cancer free. Tumors can live deep inside the gland and not raise a lump on the surface."

Another problem is that many cancers are multifocal. There may be as many as seven or more small colonies in various parts of the prostate. A small colony may not be palpable. Before we had the PSA blood test many prostate cancers were not detected by DRE. A DRE requires a lot of skill, practice and a very sensitive finger. At a presentation to a UCLA support group, a doctor used a copy of Michelangelo's famous Sistine Chapel painting where God is reaching forth with his finger and touching Adam's finger. Not many urologists have a finger that's been touched by God, but many of them are very good. Most men get their annual checkup from a family physician who may not have the skill and sensitive finger of

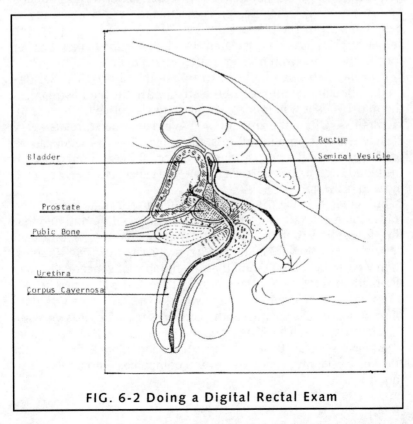

FIG. 6-2 Doing a Digital Rectal Exam

a good urologist. Usually, if the family physician finds anything that is a bit suspicious, the patient will be referred to a urologist.

Only the rear portion of the prostate, the peripheral zone, can be accessed and felt through the rectum. However the good news is, (if anything about cancer can be called good news), that about 70 percent of the cancers arise in this area.

Another problem is that not all men are the same. The rear portion of the prostate in some men is right against the rectal wall and is easily felt. In other men there may be up to a half inch of tissue between the rectal wall and the prostate. Another factor is that a DRE is a subjective test. If a patient with a small tumor is examined by several different doctors, each one may come to a different conclusion.

PSA TEST

Today we have an increased awareness and doctors have several methods in their armamentarium to detect and discover cancer. One of the most beneficial of the tests is the prostate specific antigen test (PSA). PSA is a protein enzyme that is normally produced by prostate cells. When semen is ejaculated, it is in a viscous or gelatinous form. The primary purpose of PSA is to help liquefy the semen after it has been ejaculated. This liquefaction makes it easier for the sperm to swim in their search for an ovum.

PSA was first used in 1979 to try to identify rapists. Besides being found in the semen, PSA is also found in the blood stream. In the mid 1980s it was found that prostate cancer cells also manufacture PSA. Often, the amount of PSA in the blood correlates very closely with the amount of prostate cancer. The PSA level can be used to monitor the progress of the cancer. If the amount of PSA in the blood stream goes up, then usually the cancer is actively spreading and growing.

But remember that the first rule about cancer is that there are no rules. Some prostate cancers become so poorly differentiated that they forget how to make PSA. Some men can have metastatic cancer with a very low PSA. But as a general rule, if the PSA doubles, then we can be fairly certain that the number of cancer cells have doubled. In some cases, the doubling time of the PSA may be just a few months or even just a few weeks. The faster the PSA doubling time, usually the faster the cancer is growing. It is very important that you have a PSA test done that can be used as a baseline. Then have several subsequent PSA tests and make a chart to plot the cancer activity. There are several companies who do PSA testing.

NORMAL PSA

When PSA was first discovered, no one knew what was normal. By checking the PSA of several thousand men, it was arbitrarily determined that the normal PSA should be between 0 and 4 nanograms per milliliter (ng/ml) of blood. (A nanogram is a billionth of a gram. It takes 28 grams to make one ounce, so a nanogram is a very small amount). We now know that several other factors are involved in what is normal and abnormal. First and foremost, all of us are different. What is normal for one man may not be for another. Some men may have significant cancer with a very low PSA. Conversely, a man may have a PSA as high as 12 ng/ml or more simply because of BPH or a prostatic infection.

Studies have also shown that PSA can be age specific and even race specific. The 4 ng/ml is not necessarily a good cutoff point for every one. If 4 ng/ml is considered normal for some younger patients, many significant cancers may be overlooked. In older men if 4 ng/ml is considered to indicate cancer, then many of them may undergo unnecessary biopsies or even have an unnecessary radical prostatectomy.

The table below is from over 200,000 men screened during Prostate Cancer Awareness Weeks (PCAWs). (The PCAW is the third week in each September. We are hoping that the whole month of September will eventually be designated for Prostate Awareness).

Any PSA greater than that listed for the age should be considered suspicious. African Americans are at a much higher risk for prostate cancer, and it is usually more aggressive when detected.

TABLE 1 AGE SPECIFIC PSA REFERENCE RANGES BY RACE

Age	White	African American	Latino	Asian
40-49	0-2.3	0-2.7	0-2.1	0-2.0
50-59	0-3.8	0-4.4	0-4.3	0-4.5
60-69	0-5.6	0-6.7	0-6.0	0-4.5
70-79	0-6.9	0-7.7	0-6.6	0-6.8

FALSE POSITIVE AND FALSE NEGATIVE PSA

PSA is one of the best biomarkers that has ever been discovered for any kind of cancer, but it is not perfect. There are several things that may cause the PSA to be elevated which might give a false indication of cancer. There are also several things that might mask the PSA and make it appear to be normal even though cancer might be present. There may be times and situations where a high level of PSA is found but there is no cancer.

Many older men have BPH which can cause a higher PSA. There are many more prostate cells if the person has enlargement due to

BPH. These extra cells may cause the PSA to be as high 10 to 15 ng/ml or more. However these high levels are the exception rather than the rule. Over 60% of men with PSA this high have prostate cancer. But the cancer cells are packed closer and tighter together and, gram for gram, a prostate cancer tumor produces 10 times more PSA than BPH tumors. In some prostate tumors there is a fairly close correlation between the volume of the cancerous tumor and the PSA. But remember, there are no rules when it comes to cancer. A man may have a small tumor, but a rather high PSA, or a large tumor and a fairly low PSA.

There are diseases such as prostatitis that can also cause a rise in PSA output. There are some prostatic disorders that are treated by prostatic massage. This can cause a temporary change in the PSA. A doctor will sometimes use a cystoscope to examine the prostate or bladder. This, and other irritations, can cause a change in the PSA output. Because of this, it is sometimes best to wait a few days after one of these procedures in order to get a more accurate PSA reading.

There are several hormones and drugs that can affect the PSA. The prostate cells utilize testosterone, but usually after it has been converted to dihydrotestosterone (DHT) by the enzyme 5 alpha-reductase. Proscar is a drug that is being used for BPH and prostate cancer. Proscar works by counteracting and inhibiting the 5 alpha-reductase. Proscar may cause the PSA to be reduced by as much as 50%. This reduction in PSA does not mean that it is curative for prostate cancer. However, some doctors believe that it can help and are using it along with hormone treatments.

A nationwide test of 18,000 men is being conducted to try to determine if Proscar can help prevent prostate cancer. The test is designed to last for ten years so we don't have any definitive data as yet.

PSA AND SEX

Normally, the little sperm would have great difficulty trying to swim in the sticky, gooey ejaculate. The PSA helps to convert the viscous ejaculate into a more liquid form a short time after ejaculation. Some studies indicate that the PSA level may go up shortly after ejaculation and remain elevated for as long as 48 hours. Other studies have failed to find an association between ejaculation and PSA elevation.

FREE PSA AND BOUND PSA

There are usually two different forms of PSA in the blood stream, the free PSA and PSA that is bound by a proteinase inhibitor. The usual PSA test measures the total PSA. Hybritech, and some other laboratories, can measure the free and bound PSA. Studies done by Dr. W.J. Catalona and others seems to indicate that if the free PSA is elevated in respect to the bound PSA, then the PSA is probably being produced by BPH. If there is a high level of bound PSA, then it is likely being manufactured by prostate cancer cells.

The free-to-bound PSA test seems to be more accurate if the PSA is BETWEEN 3—10 ng/ml. Dr. E. David Crawford, a co-author of this book, helped do a study of Free PSA (%fPSA) to Predict Prostate Cancer Probabilities.

The study was to try to determine if the percentage of free PSA to Total could held reduce unnecessary biopsies.

Cancer probabilities for %fPSA ranges were:

% Free PSA	Prostate Cancer Probability (95% Confidence Interval)
9%	(60%–80%)
9–11%	(50%–68%)
11–15%	(40%–54%)
15–20%	(29%–40%)
20–24%	(19%–30%)
24–26%	(11%–22%)
>26%	(6%–16%)

PSA VELOCITY

PSA velocity is the rate of change in PSA after several tests. If you have a PSA level that remains constant after several tests, even though it may be a bit high, then there is not much happening. But if the PSA is higher with each successive test, then you know that the cancer is growing. You should make a chart and carefully follow any change that takes place. Even if the PSA number is fairly low, if it goes up then you should become concerned. If the PSA should double, then you should become very concerned, especially, if it doubles in a fairly short time.

PROSTATE DENSITY

Quite often a man will have an enlarged prostate due to BPH along with prostate cancer. Both BPH and prostate cancer produces PSA, but prostate cancer produces about 10 times more PSA than an equivalent mass of BPH. Normally cells have spaces around them, but the cancer cells are very tightly packed up against each other. When the urologist does a DRE, he can feel the hard lumps of a tightly packed tumor. The tightly packed cells of a tumor may also show up on an ultrasound image. A urologist can determine the height, width and thickness of the prostate by using DRE and ultrasound. They can then divide the PSA number by the cubic cc of the prostate and get a fairly good idea how much of the prostate is due to BPH and how much is cancer.

OTHER TESTS

If the DRE is suspicious and the PSA test result is above normal, then the doctor may do a biopsy of the prostate. If these tests are inconclusive, or if the doctor just wants more information, there are several other tests that he may want done. Any or all of the following tests may be ordered: a bone scan, a magnetic resonance imaging (MRI) test, a computerized tomography (CT) scan, a transrectal ultrasound test (TRUS), a ploidy test, a laparoscopic test of lymph nodes, a ProstaScint test, reverse transcriptase polymerase chain reaction (RT-PCR) test and several others.

Based on the information provided by the tests, the doctor will assign a clinical stage. It is called a clinical stage because diagnosis is made in a clinical setting. The stage assigned will usually determine the treatment decision.

POST TREATMENT PSA

If a man has had surgery to remove the prostate, then his PSA should be undetectable. If the man has had radiation or cryosurgery treatment, he will probably still have some viable prostate tissue left. So it may be normal for these men to have a small amount of PSA in the blood. Recent evidence would suggest that the optimal PSA after any type of successful radiation therapy should be less than .5ng/ml or lower. The PSA should be stable from test to test. If a man has a high PSA reading after radiation or cryosurgery, and it remains high or increases in subsequent tests, then we know that all of the cancer was not killed, or that it had metastasized before treatment.

ULTRASENSITIVE PSA TEST

After a prostatectomy there should be no PSA at all because the entire prostate has been removed. If a test shows PSA, then we know that the cancer had metastasized. Metastatic cells are still prostate cancer cells, no matter whether they have set up a colony in the vertebra or lungs or wherever. These cells will continue to pour PSA into the blood stream. If a test shows that the PSA is rising after a prostatectomy, then we know that there are cancer cells still in the body somewhere.

For standard PSA tests, 0.1 to 0.2 is usually considered undetectable. The ultrasensitive tests can detect as low as 0.02 ng/ml. These tests will detect recurring PCa much sooner than a standard PSA test. If there is recurrence, early detection and treatment can help control it. At the present time there are two labs who are doing ultrasensitive testing, Quest Diagnostics at 1-800-642-4657 and Diagnostic Products at 1-800-678-6699.

The normal PSA test can only detect down to about 0.2 ng/ml.This level of accuracy is fine for pre-treatment PSA tests since there can be a wide variation due to several causes. But after treatment, especially a radical prostatectomy, there should be no PSA. Dr. Stamey et al at Stanford University devised an ultrasensitive test that may be ten times more sensitive than the normal Hybritech test. This test can show that the PSA is rising several months before it becomes high enough to be detected by the normal PSA test. If the ultrasensitive PSA test shows PSA activity, then treatments can be immediately instituted before the cancer has a chance to gain a foothold.

Below is a post from the Internet by Charles Clausen about the ultrasensitive PSA tests:

> Subj: Re: Ultra-Sensitive PSA
>
> From: cclausen@magick.net (Charles Clausen)
>
> ULTRASENSITIVE PSA ASSAYS
>
> Early PSA assays were able to reliably detect PSA levels at a detection limit only as low as about 0.4 ng./ml. In the early 90¹s when improved assays were being developed, Dr. Thomas Stamey and his associates at the Stanford University School of Medicine conducted studies of the most finely sensitive of them to determine their value in the early detection of recurrence after prostatectomy:
>
> It was concluded that ultrasensitive assays that can reliably read values in the range well below 0.1 ng./ml will detect recurrence several months and even a couple of years before the older standard assays which had a detection limit of 0.3 ng./ml. The advantage of this early detection of recurrence after prostatectomy is that further therapeutic measures such as radiation or hormone therapy may be undertaken earlier.
>
> The ultrasensitive assays are so sensitive that they will frequently detect extremely minute amounts of PSA that may be secreted by tissue cells other than prostate or prostate cancer cells, such as the urethra or the bulbo-urethral gland. Therefore an indication of very low levels of PSA detectable by these assays is not considered to be an indicator of recurrence. In some cases, even some post-RP men who are being tested with conventional assays may show a stable PSA of about 0.1 or 0.2. These men are not considered to have had recurrence unless there is an observable rise of the PSA level with three testings over a period of a few months. This criteria of three testings is applied also with the ultrasensitive assays, but the advantage is that these assays can start

defining a rising PSA at lower levels, and with greater accuracy.

The ultrasensitive assays that have been most commonly available commercially are those manufactured by Tosoh, Quest Diagnostics, and Diagnostic Products. The Diagnostic Products assay is known as the Immulite 3rd Generation, with a detection limit of 0.003 ng./ml. In 1998 Dr. Stamey said that it was the most sensitive of the assays on the market. Of interest is a DP Winter 1998 newsletter article about the assay at:

http://www.dpcweb.com/medical/cancer/articles/98_winter_psarelease.html

The Quest Diagnostics web site is: http://www.questdiagnostics.com

The Diagnostic Products web site is: http://www.dpcweb.com

The Tosoh PSA web page is: http://www.tosohm.com/html/tosoh_psa.html

These web sites may be helpful in locating local labs which offer the assays.

A SIMPLE PSA TEST

The Biosafe Company has developed a very simple PSA test that uses just a couple drops of blood from a pin prick of a finger. It is somewhat similar to the diabetes tests. The Biosafe company provides a home kit with all that is needed to collect the blood then send it to their lab. It could be a very good tool for prostate screening. A lot of people would submit to a finger stick at home rather than having to draw a vial of blood with a large needle.

At this time, they can only detect PSA between 0.6 and 10. This would be good enough for men who have not been treated. They are developing a more sensitive test.

You can order the kit from their web site at http://www.psa4.com orwrite to them at Biosafe Laboratories, 8600 W. Catalpa Ave., Chicago, IL 60656-9907 Tel. 1-888-700-8378

The Qualisys Diagnostics Company has a simple PSA test device called the FastPack System. It is a small device that sits on the desk. The machine is 13 inches wide, 9 inches high and 12 inches deep. A blood sample is placed in the machine and within fifteen minutes you have the results. It uses the chemiluminescence assay and performs a broad range of tests.

The company is located in Carlsbad, California—Phone 760-918-9165. They have a website at www.qualisysdiagnostics.com

PSA GRAPH

The PSA correlates fairly closely with the prostate cancer activity. It would be wise to have three or more PSA tests and track the trend before you have a major treatment. If it begins to go up, then you should be concerned.

John Fistere is a computer programming whiz. He has written a program called MultiGraph that will construct a graph for you showing the trends of your disease. All you have to do is send him a digest of your history by email. It's a free service of the Prostate Cancer Research and Education Foundation (PCREF). Send a message to John at JFistere@email.msn.com for instructions. John has contributed greatly to the fight against prostate cancer.

TRANSRECTAL ULTRASOUND

Many prostate cancers can be seen with ultrasound using a special rectal probe that is inserted into the rectum. This is called transrectal ultrasound or TRUS. Cancer tumors are usually much more dense than normal tissue. There are many different types of cancers. Rather than being a lump, the tumor may have an irregular surface and exhibit extensions of the cancer into nearby tissues.

Of course, a DRE should be done to see if there are any abnormalities that can be felt. Using DRE, PSA and TRUS, almost all prostate cancers can be detected. There are ultrasound machines that use a color Doppler effect that can be very effective in seeing cancers. One of the features of cancer is that they are usually highly vascular. The Doppler systems can see the blood vessels in color. One of the disadvantages is that these machines are very expensive.

ARTIFICIAL NEURAL NETWORK ANALYSIS (ANNA)

Drs. Crawford, Loch and others have evaluated the use of artificial intelligence to aid in the interpretation of ultrasound images and have found that this technique may be useful in determining the presence of cancer.

A portion of the 1994 PCAW database was used to train an artificial neural network. The database consisted of 39 clinical and demographic variables gathered on patients throughout the United States. The neural network was designed to diagnose the presence or absence of CaP. The portion of the database used by the neural network consisted of 1500 men all of whom had either an elevated PSA level or a suspicious digital rectal examination. These men all underwent a biopsy to confirm the presence of prostate cancer. Seventy-five percent of this group had a negative biopsy. An artificial neural network was trained and tested using 90% of this database. The remaining 10% was used in a prospective sense to validate the predictive ability of the network.

ANNA blindly classified 378 (99%) of the 381 confirmed benign pathology-confirmed samples correctly as true negatives. The false positive rate was 1% (n = 3). Of the 119 pathology-confirmed malignant samples, 94 (79%) were classified correctly; 25 (21%) were falsely classified as negatives. Of all 119 cancers, ANNA classified 60 (71%) of the hypoechoic cancers as cancers and 24 (29%) as false negatives. Surprisingly, 34 (97%) of the isoechoic cancers were correctly classified by the ANNA, missing only 1 sample. Pathologic tumor stage was correctly determined preoperative by TRUS in 52% and by 3D-ANNA in 82%. TRUS underestimated tumor stage in 40%, 3D-ANNA in 18% of the cases.

The introduction of 3D-ANNA significantly increases the accuracy of prostate cancer detection and staging. The ability to differentiate among non visible isoechoic cancerous lesions appears to be promising, and is an improvement over conventional TRUS.

BIOPSY

A biopsy is one of the better ways to determine if cancer is present. It is a very important test. A hollow needle is usually inserted into the prostate with the intent of penetrating the cancer. The needle picks up a small core of the prostate which is then examined under a microscope by a pathologist for cancerous cells. We have devoted the entire next chapter to biopsies and pathology.

Many cancers are multifocal, that is there may be several small colonies in the prostate. Remember also that the word cancer means crab, so it may have several extensions or "legs." It is possible that some or all of the cancer will be missed. The biopsy may be a hit or miss procedure. Some doctors, such as Dr. Fred Lee at Crittendon Hospital, use a color Doppler Transurethral Ultrasound (TRUS) to find the cancer. He has had great success.

GLEASON SCORE

Prostate cancer cells may not all be the same. A colony may be much like a family, with some very young cells that are just starting to become cancerous, some that are in the intermediate stage, and some that are old.The younger ones may look very much like a normal cell, or well differentiated. (The term differentiated is derived from the embryo which develops from the original egg and sperm. All subsequent growth is due to cells that become different or differentiate into arms, legs, muscles and all of the other tissues of our body). The intermediate cancer cells may be somewhat changed and moderately differentiated, while the older ones may be very much changed and poorly differentiated. Those that are poorly differentiated are usually more aggressive and subject to metastasis.

Dr. D.F. Gleason was a pathologist who specialized in prostate cancer. He determined that there could be five different types of prostate cancer cells. Depending on the differentiation of the cells, he graded them from I to V. If he looked in the microscope and saw a large number of cells that were well differentiated, he might call them a grade 1. If there was another group that was less differentiated, he might call it a grade 2. If they were moderately differentiated, he might give them a grade of 3. If some of the cells were poorly differentiated, he might call them a grade 4. The really bad ones were assigned a grade 5. The grades of the two types of cells that were most prevalent were then added to give a final score. In the instance above, the 3 and 4 would be added for a score of seven. The first figure indicates the greatest number of that type so the example above would indicate more type 3 than type 4. If the figures were 4 plus 3, it would mean that there was more grade 4 than 3. This would indicate a worse prognosis. Figure 6-1 shows a copy of Dr. Gleason's drawing.

A low-grade tumor might be one that has a Gleason score of 2, 3, or 4. A medium grade would have a Gleason score of 5, 6 or 7. A high-grade tumor would be one that has a Gleason score of 8, 9, or 10. Ordinarily, if the Gleason score is 5 or less, the cancer may not need treatment except to watch and wait. A Gleason score of 6 or 7 should be cause for concern. If either one of the individual scores is 4 or more there is cause for concern. A score of 8, 9, or 10 usually indicates a very aggressive cancer. These cancers have probably metastasized, are usually systemic and may have a poor prognosis.

Since the Gleason score is subjective to some extent, usually two or more pathologists will examine the sample.

PLOIDY TESTS

A ploidy test is another test that tries to determine the aggressiveness of the cancer. All of our normal cells are diploid, that is they have two identical sets, or 23 pairs, of chromosomes in the nucleus. A cancer cell may be aneuploid which means that it may have an uneven number of chromosomes. The cell may also be tetraploid, with four sets or polyploid with a large number of sets.

The ploidy test measures the amount of DNA in the cells. If there is an abnormal amount, then the cells are more likely to be aggressive. The test can often be done from tissue removed during biopsy. The ploidy test is rather expensive. Some doctors do not believe that it is worthwhile.

Here is a post on the internet about ploidy by John Fistere:

> "I went to a lecture at our support group titled 'Understanding the DNA Ploidy Test', given by Perrin McDaniel, General Manager, Cytometry Associates. Surprisingly, I now understand the DNA ploidy test:-) (an Internet grin). The test simply measures the amount of DNA in cells as they flow past a certain point. The cells have been stained with a dye that fluoresces only when bound to DNA. The results are displayed on a chart that effectively has a percentage of cells on the vertical scale, and brightness, or amount of DNA, on the horizontal scale. If all the cells were normal, and 'at rest' (diploid) then there would be one peak on the chart, corresponding to the amount of DNA in a normal cell.
>
> "However not all cells are at rest. Some are "ready" to divide. These cells will show as a second peak at about twice the brightness, because they have synthesized a second set of chromosomes in preparation for mitosis, or cell division. These cells are tetraploid, but normal. Typically that peak will be no more that 15% of the cell population (or maybe it was 15% of the main peak). Some cells are in the process of synthesizing DNA to get ready for division, so they will show up somewhere in between the diploid and tetraploid, and will not have a peak. So, for a population of normal cells you have two peaks, with a level in between.
>
> "What can happen is that abnormal cells will develop with different chromosome complements, usually more than diploid, and they will continue to multiply with that abnormal amount of DNA, and produce a peak on the chart at some other location. The population of cells that produce that peak is sometimes called a "cell line". Also, if the tetraploid peak is too high, above the arbitrary 15% limit, it indicates that there are abnormal tetraploid cells in the population. Although I have not studied ploidy reports, the speaker indicated that the report would state whether or not there was an aneuploid population, and report the percentage of cells 1) at rest, 2) synthesizing DNA and 3) ready to divide. He did not say so, but I would think the report would include the percentage of aneuploid cells in the sample."

Dr. Jonathan Oppenheimer says that he, and many other pathologists, can make a fairly good estimation of the ploidy by just looking at the slides from a biopsy to determine the Gleason. He says his estimations correlate rather well with the laboratory flow cytometry tests. (And his estimations are a lot less expensive than the lab tests). You might ask if your pathologist can do the same. At the present time, the value of the ploidy testing is controversial. One of the problems relates to sampling errors from the biopsy.

BONE SCAN

If the prostate cancer has metastasized, it often sets up colonies in the bones. Without a good blood supply, a tumor is severely limited in how large it can grow. The bone marrow is very rich in blood so the cells can readily establish colonies. These colonies can be seen with an X-ray bone scan.

To do a bone scan, a radionuclide substance is injected into the patient. The radioactive substance will seek out bone cancer and will show up on an x-ray as a "hot spot." Some doctors do a bone scan routinely, but in many cases it is not needed. Several studies have shown that if the PSA is less than 10 ng/ml and the Gleason score is less than seven the bone scan will be negative in all but a very few cases. Because of HMO and insurance restrictions, the doctors are now more selective in recommending a bone scan.

REVERSE TRANSCRIPTASE POLYMERASE CHAIN REACTION

Reverse Transcriptase Polymerase Chain Reaction (RT-PCR) is a very sensitive DNA test that can detect just a few prostate cancer cells in the blood stream. Finding a cancer cell in the blood stream before treatment might indicate that the cancer has escaped the prostate and has already metastasized. If the cancer has already metastasized, then it won't help much to remove the prostate. But it is rather difficult for a cancer cell to establish a new colony. It must find a good site and establish new blood vessel. While doing this, the cancer cell must avoid being recognized and destroyed by the body's defenses.

Dr. Michael Sokoloff et al at UCLA did a study that was reported in the November 1996 issue of the Journal of Urology. This study found…"Circulating PSA producing cells were present in 29 of 33 patients(88%) with metastatic prostate cancer. Two of 19 patients (11%) with no known prostate cancer exhibited positive signals (1 later had PCa).

Positive PSA polymerase chain reactions were detected in 30 of 51 patients (59%) with stages pT1 and pT2 disease and in 13 of 18 (72%) with stage pT3 cancer. No significant relationship of a positive PSA PCR signal to pathologic stage, tumor grade, apical involvement or positive surgical margins was found…

Conclusions: in patients with pathologically determined localized disease, in our experience PCR based assays offer no immediate benefit for preoperative staging…"

Of course if the patient has had a prostatectomy and a RT-PCR test finds prostate cancer cells in the blood-stream, then the patient has metastatic cancer.

PROSTASCINT

ProstaScint is approved as a diagnostic imaging agent in newly diagnosed patients with biopsy proven prostate cancer who may be at high risk for pelvic lymph node metastases. ProstaScint is also indicated as a diagnostic imaging agent in post-prostatectomy patients with a rising PSA and a negative or equivocal standard metastatic evaluation in whom there is a high clinical suspicion of occult metastatic disease.

The ProstaScint test uses monoclonal antibodies that are specific to prostate cancer.

The antibodies are designed specifically to detect cancer in soft tissues. The antibody is combined with a radioactive tracer, Indium 111, to create a substance that is injected into the patient's system. The antibody then attaches itself to the walls of prostate cancer cells and, with the aid of a radioactive tracer, a scan reveals the location of the cancer.

The antibodies have an affinity for prostate cells, so most will search out those cells and settle there. The body is then scanned with a gamma ray camera which can locate the radioactive antibodies and metastatic areas. A gamma ray camera is similar to a geiger counter which can detect radioactive rays.

In post-prostatectomy patients who have a rising PSA, ProstaScint scans can distinguish between cancer which has recurred at the previous site of surgery and cancer which has spread either regionally or distantly. This additional staging information may be helpful in selecting the most appropriate therapy for you.

Sometimes cancer will spread to bone. A radionuclide bone scan is able to detect metastases. However, a bone scan will not detect metastases in soft tissue (e.g. the lymph nodes). In contrast, a ProstaScint scan can detect cancer that has spread to the lymph nodes, and, although it may sometimes identify bony metastases, it is much less sensitive than a bone scan. Consequently both tests may sometimes be needed.

A disadvantage of the ProstaScint test is that it is rather expensive. It may also be difficult to interpret the test results. There may be false positives and false negatives. Only about 70% of the tests are accurate.

The ProstaScint imaging study provides prognostic information which complements other diagnostic indicators in cases of prostate cancer where there is a high clinical suspicion of metastasis. Because it requires specific training for optimal administration and interpretation, CYTOGEN has established a growing network of non-affilitated imaging centers where personnel have undertaken this specific training.

For more information visithttp://www.prostascint.com or www.cytogen.com

Cytogen provides a list of several centers, by state, where one can get a ProstaScint test. Go to: http://www.prostascint.com/pie_dir_mstr.jsp

Tel: 609-987-8200
Fax: 609-987-6450
Email: imaging@cytogen.com

MICROMETASTASES

Despite all the tests that may be performed, there is still the possibility that some of the cells may have escaped the prostate and formed a micrometastatic colony somewhere in the body. It would be impossible to detect a small colony of just a few cells. If it is a fairly large colony, the ProstaScint test will probably detect it. And of course, if it is a fairly large colony that has set up in the bones, a bone scan will detect it.

LYMPHADENECTOMY

When the cancer escapes the prostate, it will often be found in the pelvic lymph nodes. When a radical prostatectomy is performed, usually one of the first things done after opening the man is to check the lymph nodes. They send them out to be quick frozen and checked for cancer cells. If cancer is present in the lymph nodes, the operation is usually halted. It wouldn't do much good to remove the prostate if the cancer is systemic.

If the man is going to have brachytherapy or seed implants, or other forms of radiation, proton beam therapy or cryosurgery, there will be no opportunity to check the lymph nodes. Some doctors have advised that if any of the patients considering these therapies have a PSA greater than 20 ng/ml or a Gleason Score of 7 or more, then it might be worthwhile to have a pelvic laparoscopic lymphadenectomy. The laparoscope is a small tubular instrument with lenses and several attachments. It can be inserted into the abdomen or pelvic area to harvest lymph nodes. If a harvested lymph node proves to be positive for cancer cells, then more appropriate treatments should be considered.

Dr. Crawford and others have set up an artificial Intelligence System that can be used to predict lymph node involvement and save a lot of unnecessary lymphadenectomies. Approximately 125,000 radical prostatectomies are performed annually as treatment for prostate cancer in the US. Only 5 to10% of patients that have lymphadenectomy with radical prostatectomy have pathology proven lymph node disease. Therefore, approximately 90-95% of these lymphadenectomies are unnecessary.

A database of 4,133 patient records was used to train and validate the AI system. Using this technology, we can identify patients at low risk for lymph node involvement with an accuracy of 98-99% and thereby avoid performing unnecessary lymphadenectomies on these patients.

STAGING SYSTEMS

Once all the tests have been done and as much information as possible has been gathered, the doctor will then assign a clinical stage (CS). Of course the clinical stage may not be completely accurate. The only way to be absolutely sure of a stage is to remove the prostate and have a pathologist examine it. Even then, it is possible that the man may have micrometastases somewhere that would not show up on any test that we have.

For several years, urologists have used the Whitmore-Jewett staging system of A, B, C and D. Each of these main stages had substages that helped to better describe the tumor. But there are some instances where this system does not give enough information about the disease. Many doctors and publications are now switching to a Tumor-Node-Metastases (TNM) system.

The Whitmore-Jewett system (stages A through D) was described in 1975 and has since been modified. In 1997, the American Joint Committee on Cancer (AJCC) and the International Union Against Cancer, adopted a revised TNM system which employs the same broad T stage categories as the Whitmore-Jewett system. But it includes subcategories of T stage, including a stage to describe patients diagnosed through PSA screening. This revised TNM system is clinically useful and more precisely stratifies newly diagnosed patients. Both staging systems are shown below.

TNM definitions

Primary tumor (T)

TX: Primary tumor cannot be assessed

T0: No evidence of primary tumor

T1a: Tumor incidental histologic finding in 5% or less of tissue resected in TURP

T1b: Tumor incidental histologic finding in more than 5% of tissue resected in TURP

T1c: Tumor identified by needle biopsy (e.g., because of elevated PSA)

T2a: Tumor involves 1 lobe

T2b: Tumor involves both lobes

T3a: Extracapsular extension (unilateral or bilateral)

T3b: Tumor invades seminal vesicle(s)

T3c: Cancer that has invaded the seminal vesicles

T4a: Tumor that involves the bladder neck and/or external sphincter and/or rectum

T4b: Cancer that involves other pelvic areas near the prostate

N0: No cancer detected in the lymph nodes

N1 (N+): Cancer spread to one or more lymph nodes (2 cm of cancer or less)

N2 (N+): Cancer spread to one or more lymph nodes (2cm to 5 cm of cancer)

N3 (N+): Cancer spread to one or more lymph nodes (5cm of cancer or more)

M0: No distant metastasis

M1 (M+) Distant metastases

Histopathologic grade (G)

GX: Grade cannot be assessed

G1: Well differentiated (slight anaplasia)

G2: Moderately differentiated (moderate anaplasia)

G3-4: Poorly differentiated or undifferentiated (marked anaplasia)

AJCC stage groupings

Stage I

T1a, N0, M0, G1

Stage II

T1a, N0, M0, G2, 3-4

T1b, N0, M0, Any G

T1c, N0, M0, Any G

T1, N0, M0, Any G

T2, N0, M0, Any G

Stage III

T3, N0, M0, Any G

Stage IV

T4, N0, M0, Any G

Any T, N1, M0, Any G

Any T, Any N, M1, Any G

The Whitmore-Jewett staging system is as described below:

A1: Clinically undetectable tumor confined to the prostate gland and is an incidental finding at prostatic surgery such as a TURP. Same as T1a, less than 5% of prostate.

A2: Unsuspected tumor found during a TURP, same as T1b, occupies more than 5%

B1: Cancer that is felt—may occupy 50% or more of one side, same as T2a

B2: Cancer that is felt and occupies both sides of prostate, Same as T2b

C1: Cancer that is growing outside the prostate, one or both sides, same as T3a

C2: Cancer that has invaded the seminal vesicles and/or the bladder neck, same as T3c, rectum and other nearby pelvic areas, same as T4a

D1: Cancer that has spread to one or more lymph nodes, same as T4b

D2: Cancer that has spread and set up distant metastases

D3: D2 prostate cancer patients who relapsed after adequate endocrine therapy

Figure 6-3 shows a drawing of a normal prostate. Fig. 6-4 shows a stage T 1 or A, fig. 6-5 shows a stage T2 or B, fig. 6-6 shows a stage T3 or C and fig. 6-7 shows a stage D. (These drawings are courtesy of the Schering Company).

One of the co-authors of this book, Dr. E. David Crawford, has suggested that the D stage should have further categories. It is important to classify patients with advanced prostate cancer by evaluating the actual behavior of the disease. Not all patients with advancing disease are stage D1 or D2. There are an increasing number of patients with stage D1.5 disease. This subset of patients are identified as having a small tumor burden and a rising PSA after failing local therapy.

Another important subset of patients are those who successfully received hormonal manipulation and later had a rising PSA. These patients should be classified as stage D2.5, which is becoming the most frequent presentation of advanced disease. The benefit of further separating the hormone sensitive from the hormone insensitive patient is that it selects cohorts that may benefit from earlier chemotherapeutic efforts.

GRADE VS. STAGE

A Gleason Grade (GG) is used to designate each of the individual components that make up the Gleason Score (GS). For instance a biopsy might contain Gleason Grade 3 as the primary component

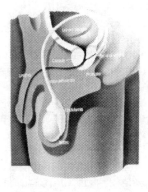

FIG. 6-3 A Normal Prostate

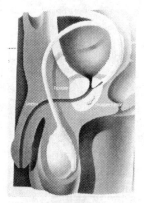

FIG. 6-4 A Stage T1 or A Tumor

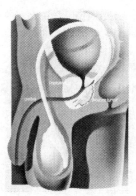

FIG. 6-5 A Stage T2 or B Tumor

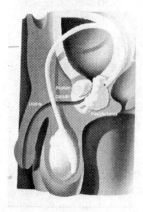

FIG. 6-6 A Stage T3 or C Tumor

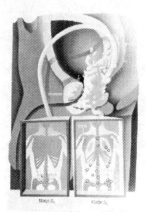

6-7 Stage D Tumor

and a Gleason Grade 4 as the secondary component. This would give a Gleason Score of 7.

Grade and stage are sometimes confused. Prostate cancer has been arbitrarily divided into three grades of disease. A man with a Gleason score of 2, 3 and 4 would be considered have a Grade 1 disease; a Gleason score of 5, 6 and 7 would be Grade 2 disease; and a Gleason score of 8, 9 and 10 would be Grade 3 disease. They are also designated as low grade, medium grade and high grade.

Dr. Jonathan Oppenheimer is a pathologist. He doesn't like these designations. Many doctors consider any Gleason grade that has a 4 component such as 4+3 or even 2+4 should be considered to be high grade or at least Grade 2. (Grade 2+4 is unusual, but my friend Ralph Valle had this score). Dr. Oppenheimer said that the person who decided this grading system should be given a DRE with a hot jalapeno pepper.

Knowing the PSA, the Gleason Score and the clinical stage and the Partin/Narayan Tables predictions, can help the doctor and you to choose the best form of treatment.

MAGNETIC RESONANCE IMAGING AND MAGNETIC RESONANCE SPECTROGRAPHIC IMAGING (MRI/MRSI)

Fig. 6-10 shows a MRI machine and a diagram. Here is a bit of information about Magnetic Resonance Imaging (MRI) and Magnetic Resonance Spectrographic Imaging (MRSI):

MR imaging emerged in 1980 as an outgrowth of the use of nuclear magnetic resonance to study the structure of chemical compounds. MR imaging has several advantages over conventional radiography:

- It does not use ionizing radiation, so it is safer than conventional radiography or CT.
- It can obtain images in sagittal, coronal, transverse, and/or oblique planes.
- The endorectal/pelvic phased coil MRI is highly accurate in detecting seminal vesicle invasion and extracapsular extension of prostate cancer (96% and 81%, respectively).
- Within the same exam, MRI can also be used to assess cancer that has spread to the pelvic lymph nodes or bone.

However, even with all of these advantages, the MRI has limitations:

- Localization of cancer within the prostate is subject to error because of factors such as post-biopsy hemorrhage, chronic prostatitis, BPH, intraglandular dysplasia, trauma, and therapy. This can lead to an overestimation of the spatial extent of cancer and extracapsular extension.

- MRI alone has demonstrated a high sensitivity but low specificity in determining tumor location within the gland due to a large number of false positives. But the combined MRI/MRSI study provides high resolution anatomic imaging and nuclear magnetic resonance spectroscopy data. The result is that one can observe specific resonances (peaks) for citrate, choline and creatine from 0.24cc volumes throughout the gland. The area under these peaks is related to the concentration of these metabolites and changes in these concentrations can be used to identify cancer.

Dr. Joseph P. Hornak has an excellent web site called the Basics of MRI at http://www.cis.rit.edu/htbooks/mri/inside.htm

It is a complete book that you can read online. It is a bit technical and may tell you more about MRI than you want to know.

Here is a short article on MRI by Bernie Beskind, e-mail bernieb@CITYWORLD.COM:

I just returned from getting my MRI/MRSI at UCSF, and thought I would document the test, the content of my report, and my experiences with the staff, facility and area.

THE MRI/MRSI TEST (Condensed from the UCSF Patient Manual)

While both tests are FDA approved, the accuracy of the combined magnetic resonance imaging (MRI) and magnetic resonance spectroscopic imaging (MRSI) for assessing the presence and spatial extent of prostate cancer is still undergoing clinical investigation. MRI uses a strong magnetic field and radio frequency waves to non-invasively obtain anatomic pictures based on tissue water.

MRSI creates a metabolic picture based on the relative concentrations of the cellular metabolites citrate, creatine and choline. The area under the peak returns from these substances is related to the concentrations of these metabolites, and changes in these concentrations can be used to identify cancer. To date, over 2000 prostate cancer patients have been studied using this combined exam. In a study of 62 patients who had the exam prior to an RP followed by step-section histopathology, it was demonstrated the prostate cancer could be localized to a sextant of the prostate with a specificity of up to 91% when both were positive for cancer, and a sensitivity of up to 95% when either were positive for cancer.(My note:I think this means that when both are positive, it is 91% correct that cancer is present, and when both are negative, it is 95% correct that cancer is absent.)The test is especially appropriate for determining extracapsular extension and seminal vesicle invasion. It is less accurate for assessing lymph node invasion. It can help guide treatment decisions and assess a post treatment rising PSA.

The test takes about an hour. The patient is on a light diet the day before and the day of the treatment, and takes a Fleet enema 1-3 hours prior. I did not see the probe, but was told it is slightly larger than an ultrasound probe. Depending on your trunk length (pelvis to head), you may not be completely engulfed by the MRI machine (my eyes could see the edge of the apparatus.)Your body is strapped down to limit movement, and a heavy flat plate is placed on your pelvis and abdomen. I assumed that must contain some recording film.

Inserting the probe was very uncomfortable, but the (male) nurse was very gentle, took his time, and told me at the outset what to expect and emphasized that I was in charge. He would stop whenever I gave the word. I did not have to do so. Once the probe was in place, I had no discomfort or even awareness of it being there. They offered ear phones with music, but with the risk of going asleep which would invalidate the results. I wore soft ear plugs instead, and kept time to the jack hammers.:-)

MY TEST REPORT: Gave my prostate volume and PSA density. Noted a mildly thickened bladder wall, suggesting a degree of outlet obstruction. Showed no post-biopsy hemorrhage. Stated that "areas of reduced T2 signal in the peripheral zone of the (RIGHT mid gland to apex) may represent tumor." Stated that "MRSI demonstrates several voxels (in RIGHT mid gland to apex) of positive and possible malignant metabolism." The two images indicate a moderate volume of tumor dominant in the RIGHT mid gland to apex. Noted minimal capsular irregularity on a single image at the right apex is of questionable significance, and not considered...to indicate extra-capsular extension. (NOTE—one surgeon noted a "hardness" on the right side during a DRE.) Stated that no other sites of ECE, nor any SVI, lymphadenopathy or suspicious bone lesion seen.

This information was a major element in my treatment decision. The test was well worth the trip, money and inconvenience.

Editorial Note: Based on the above tests and other investigations, Bernie decided to have the High Dose Rate (HDR) temporary seed implants. It was done at the Long Beach Memorial Hospital by Dr. Nisar Syed. Bernie is doing fine.

To contact the Magnetic Resonance Science Center, University of California San Francisco Medical Center, telephone (415) 476-9023.

Here is a web site that has a complete book about MRI online called:

ELEMENTARY FUNCTIONAL MRI DATA ANALYSIS: A USER'S MANUAL

http://www.nmr.mgh.harvard.edu/fmrianalysis/index.html

There is a web site for Clinical Magnetic Resonance Society at http://www.cmrs.com/benefits.html

You can find a directory of MRI sites at http://www.healthimaging.com
There are several other MRI sites in this country and in foreign countries. Search the Internet for more locations.

ULTRASOUND COLOR DOPPLER

Ultrasound Color Doppler can be a very good diagnostic tool. Prostate cancer has increased vascularity. Blood flow is detected by Doppler frequency shifts, and displayed as a color overlay on the image.

Dr. Fred Lee at Crittendon Hospital in Grand Rapids Michigan is one of the experts at using ultrasound color Doppler. Read more about him at:

http://www.prostatepointers.org/prostate/lee/small/lee1.html
There is some excellent information and beautiful color Doppler photos at:

http://prostate.tju.edu/ultrasound/color.html

RECURRENCE

Even when caught early and with the best treatment, there is no guarantee that prostate cancer will not recur. About 20% of the men who undergo radical prostatectomies, brachytherapy, radiation and other definitive treatments have a recurrence within 5 years. In some cases, a small micrometastasis colony had already been established somewhere in the body before treatment.

Dr. E. David Crawford and others have been investigating the use of artificial neural network analysis (ANNA) for the prediction of prostate cancer recurrence. Overall accuracy was 85%. A pattern exists in our data which allows the neural network to give predictive values for pathological staging between 75% and 80%. The variables in order of importance were Gleason primary score, biopsy stage, Gleason sum, DRE, original PSA, prostate volume, and prior therapy whether radiation or hormonal manipulation.

TREATMENTS FOR RECURRENCE

There are several treatments that can be used if the cancer recurs. External beam radiation can be used if it is determined that the recurrence is local. If it is a distant metastasis, then hormone therapy or possibly chemotherapy may be the treatment of choice.

PSA, STAGE & GLEASON SCORE

The PSA and Gleason score may be different for different stages. It is possible to have a low PSA with a stage T2b tumor but have a Gleason score of 8 or 9. It is also possible to have a high PSA with a stage T2b tumor and a Gleason score of 5 or 6. Ordinarily, a high Gleason score is more important than the PSA and the stage. Having a low stage such as T1b is no guarantee that the cancer will not metastasize. One study done at the Long Beach Memorial Hospital by Drs. Nisar Syed and Ajmel Puthawala showed that out of 32 patients diagnosed with T1b disease, four of them progressed to metastasis within five years, or 12 percent of the patients. In the same group of patients, 85 had T2b disease. Only seven, or 8 percent of these T2b patients progressed to metastasis within five years. Again, the first rule in cancer is that there are no rules. What may seem like an indolent or insignificant disease may very well become incurable.

THE PARTIN/NARAYAN TABLES

Before a treatment decision is made, there are a couple more tools that should be utilized. They are the Partin and Narayan Tables. The Partin Tables, (see Tables 6-1 to 6-4) were developed by Dr. Alan Partin, and several other urologists at Johns Hopkins University and are based on data from over 500 radical prostatectomies that had been done. Dr. Alan Partin of Johns Hopkins did a retrospective study of the men who had undergone a radical prostatectomy. Using the data in the case histories, he constructed the Partin Tables. Once a stage has been assigned, your PSA established, and you know your Gleason score from the biopsy, you can look at these tables and get a good idea of what the odds are that you have an organ confined disease (OCD), Extra Capsular Extension (ECE), seminal vesicle invasion (SVI), or positive lymph nodes. Later Dr. Partin looked at case histories of over 5000 men. This much larger group of men gives the Tables a lot more confidence.

Dr. Narayan devised a slightly different table than Dr. Partin's. Dr. Stephen Strum combined the two to give a more accurate prediction. Dr. Glenn Tisman, who worked with Dr. Strum, created a computer program that can automatically calculate your risks after you key in your PSA, stage and Gleason. You can find these tables and several other papers by Dr. Stephen Strum at www.prostatepointers.org/80/strum/.

Using your assigned stage, your PSA, and Gleason score, you can predict the percentage of the probability of localized organ confinement, capsular penetration, seminal vesicle involvement, and lymph node involvement.

Knowing the odds of the various involvements should greatly influence your treatment decision.

Comparison of PSA, Gleason's Score & Clinical Stage per Partin+
vs PSA, GS, TRUSP stage per Narayan*

- Prediction of organ-confined Disease
- Prediction of extra-capsular extension
- Prediction of lymph node involvement
- Prediction of seminal vesicle involvement

Prediction of organ-confined Disease

GS	Clinical stages according to Partin et al & Narayan et al (see legend**)								
	T1a	T1b	T1c	T2a	T2b	B1	T2c	B2	T3a
2-4	100	85	92	88	76	90	82	86	-
5	100	78	81	81	67	87	73	82	-
6	100	68	69	72	54	84	60	69	42
7	-	54	55	61	41	78	46	67	-
8-10	-	-	-	48	31	72	-	60	-
For PSA values up to 4.0 use table section above									
2-4	100	78	82	83	67	89	71	82	-
5	100	70	71	73	56	85	64	78	43
6	100	53	59	62	44	81	48	66	33
7	100	39	43	51	32	75	37	61	26
8-10	-	32	31	39	22	69	25	55	12
For PSA values 4.1-10 use table section above									
2-4	100	-	-	61	52	82	-	78	-
5	100	49	55	58	43	77	37	68	26
6	-	36	41	44	28	70	37	53	19
7	-	24	24	36	19	63	24	49	14
8-10	-	11	-	29	14	60	15	41	9
For PSA values 10.1-20 use table section above									
2-4	-	-	33	20	7	75	-	64	-
5	-	-	24	32	-	65	3	56	-
6	-	-	22	14	11	59	4	41	5
7	-	-	7	18	4	45	5	20	3
8-10	-	-	3	3	1	42	2	13	2
For PSA values greater than 20 use table section above									
** B1 of Narayan is combination of stages T2a + T2b of Partin									
B2 of Narayan is equivalent of T2c of Partin									
All numbers in bold are from Narayan paper; remainder from Partin paper									
Narayan numbers from 4.1-10, 10.1-20 are approximations from graph									

Table **6-1** Partin-Narayan

Prediction of extra-capsular extension(Narayan) and Capsular Penetration (Partin)

GS	Clinical stages according to Partin et al & Narayan et al (see legend)								
	T1a	T1b	T1c	T2a	T2b	B1	T2c	B2	T3a
2-4	0	15	22	14	26	10	17	14	-
5	0	22	30	20	34	13	26	17	-
6	0	30	34	29	46	16	38	21	59
7	-	43	40	39	59	20	50	27	-
8-10	-	-	-	50	68	24	-	33	-
For PSA values up to 4.0 use table section above									
2-4	0	22	29	19	34	11	27	15	-
5	0	29	34	28	45	14	34	20	58
6	0	45	38	38	56	17	49	25	68
7	0	58	44	49	68	22	59	31	75
8-10	-	64	48	59	77	26	71	36	87
For PSA values 4.1-10 use table section above									
2-4	0	-	-	40	49	14	-	37	-
5	0	49	40	43	58	18	61	45	75
6	-	62	45	56	73	22	59	53	82
7	-	73	52	64	81	27	73	60	86
8-10	-	87	-	70	86	32	82	66	92
For PSA values 10.1-20 use table section above									
2-4	-	-	50	80	94	20	-	37	-
5	-	-	54	68	-	24	97	45	-
6	-	-	53	86	90	28	96	53	95
7	-	-	67	80	96	35	95	60	98
8-10	-	-	74	97	99	41	97	66	98
For PSA values greater than 20 use table section above									
** B1 of Narayan is combination of stages T2a + T2b of Partin									
B2 of Narayan is equivalent of T2c of Partin									
All numbers in bold are from Narayan paper; remainder from Partin paper									
Narayan numbers from 4.1-10, 10.1-20 are approximations from graph									

Table **6**-2 Partin-Narayan

Prediction of Lymph Node Involvement

GS	Clinical stages according to Partin et al & Narayan et al (see legend)								
	T1a	T1b	T1c	T2a	T2b	B1	T2c	B2	T3a
2-4	0	2	<1	1	2	1	4	2	-
5	0	4	1	2	4	2	9	2	-
6	0	8	2	3	9	2	17	2	15
7	-	15	2	7	18	2	31	10	-
8-10	-	-	-	13	32	3	-	16	-
For PSA values up to 4.0 use table section above									
2-4	0	2	1	1	2	1	5	1	-
5	0	4	1	2	5	1	10	1	8
6	0	9	2	4	11	3	19	1	16
7	0	18	3	8	20	3	34	12	28
8-10	0	30	5	15	35	4	53	20	50
For PSA values 4.1-10 use table section above									
2-4	0	-	-	1	3	3	-	6	-
5	0	5	3	2	6	4	13	10	11
6	-	11	4	5	13	6	22	16	20
7	-	21	7	9	24	8	39	25	35
8-10	-	41	-	17	40	11	59	37	54
For PSA values 10.1-20 use table section above									
2-4	-	-	6	2	7	10	-	15	-
5	-	-	9	3	-	13	29	24	-
6	-	-	8	9	18	17	53	36	31
7	-	-	24	11	44	22	62	50	55
8-10	-	-	41	35	76	28	73	65	65
For PSA values greater than 20 use table section above									
** B1 of Narayan is combination of stages T2a + T2b of Partin									
B2 of Narayan is equivalent of T2c of Partin									
All numbers in bold are from Narayan paper; remainder from Partin paper									
Narayan numbers from 4.1-10, 10.1-20 are approximations from graph									

Table **6**-3 Partin-Nayaran

Prediction of Seminal Vesicle Involvement

GS	Clinical stages according to Partin et al & Narayan et al (see legend)								
	T1a	T1b	T1c	T2a	T2b	B1	T2c	B2	T3a
2-4	0	1	<1	1	2	1	2	3	-
5	0	3	<1	2	4	1	4	4	-
6	0	6	1	5	9	2	9	6	8
7	-	12	4	9	17	4	17	9	-
8-10	-	-	-	17	29	5	-	12	-
For PSA values up to 4.0 use table section above									
2-4	0	2	<1	1	3	1	3	4	-
5	0	4	<1	3	6	1	6	5	5
6	0	9	1	6	11	3	12	8	11
7	0	18	5	12	22	5	23	11	18
8-10	-	29	23	22	38	7	40	15	40
For PSA values 4.1-10 use table section above									
2-4	0	-		3	4	2	-	9	-
5	0	7	<1	5	8	4	12	11	11
6		15	1	11	19	6	17	16	18
7		28	6	19	33	10	33	21	31
8-10	-	55		29	50	15	53	29	49
For PSA values 10.1-20 use table section above									
2-4	-	-	<1	12	30	8	-	20	-
5	-	-	<1	11	-	12	29	28	-
6	-	-	2	35	40	18	53	35	31
7	-	-	9	31	73	27	62	45	55
8-10	-	-	31	81	93	38	73	55	65
For PSA values greater than 20 use table section above									
** B1 of Narayan is combination of stages T2a + T2b of Partin									
B2 of Narayan is equivalent of T2c of Partin									
All numbers in bold are from Narayan paper; remainder from Partin paper									
Narayan numbers from 4.1-10, 10.1-20 are approximations from graph									

Table 6-4 Partin-Nayaran

+ Partin AW, Yoo J, Carter CB et al: The use of prostate specific antigen, clinical stage, and Gleason score to predict pathological stage in men with localized prostate cancer. J Urol 150:110-114, 1993.

* Narayan P, Gajendran V, Taylor SP et al: The role of transrectal ultrasound-guided biopsy-based staging, preoperative serum prostate-specific antigen, and biopsy Gleason score in prediction of final pathologic diagnosis in prostate cancer. Urology 46:205-212, 1995.

GENERAL PROGNOSIS

No one can say for sure how long you will live, no matter what stage of cancer you have. If a doctor tells you that you have only so long to live, you may give up and live just that long. Studies have shown that a person who takes an active interest in his health and well-being will live much longer.

Several studies have also shown that it is important to have a social life. Men who are married live longer than those who live alone. Even if you are not married, you should join and become active in groups such as senior citizens clubs, Toastmasters, Elks, Veterans organizations or even in political organizations. Better yet is to become active in a prostate cancer support group. If there are no support groups near you, then start one. Contact US TOO at 708-323-1002 and they will tell you if there is a support group in your area. Or if you would like to start a group, they will send you a start-up kit.

We desperately need more money for prostate cancer research. We have organized a National Prostate Cancer Coalition (NPCC). We need all the help we can get. If you would like to help, contact the NPCC at 1300 19th St. N.W., #400, Washington, D.C. 20036.

Chapter Seven

WATCH AND WAIT

Drs. Aubrey Pilgrim and E. David Crawford

The word cancer can be very frightening. When some hear it, they panic and want it out immediately. But a rash decision to have a rush treatment that is not necessary may cause more problems than the cancer. In many cases, the cancer may have taken several years to grow to the point where it was detectable. It won't hurt to wait for a while so that you can investigate all your options. It could be that you may never have to have a treatment.

If you are 50 years old, and in a room with two other men, one of you probably has cancer of some kind. One out of every two men will get cancer of some kind in his lifetime. About one out of every six men may have prostate cancer during their lifetime, but many prostate cancers are latent or indolent. If you look up the word indolent it will tell you that it derives from the Latin *dolere*, to feel pain, the prefix *in*—means not, so an indolent prostate cancer would not cause pain. Indolent also means lazy or inactive. These words describe many prostate cancers. There are millions of men who have these cancers and they will never be a problem. Whether they know it or not, these men are Waiting.

Unfortunately, we have no absolute way to determine which of the cancers are truly indolent and which ones may be dangerous enough to kill you. The rate of deaths due to prostate cancer was over 40,000 per year just a short time ago. Since the advent of the PSA test the mortality figures are coming down. The estimated figure for prostate cancer deaths in 2000 was 31,900. But an autopsy is not performed on many men who die. Some men die while not under the care of a doctor. Often the real cause of death is not known. So there may be more deaths from PC than the official figures show.

Watching and Waiting may be the better option for many men. But those men who are blithely Waiting would be much better off if they were Watching closely while Waiting. One way to do this is to closely monitor the PSA.

The PSA test is one of the simplest and best markers that we have for any cancer. In most cases, the PSA will correlate fairly closely with the cancer activity. You should have a record of any PSA tests and the dates when checked. You can then check for any upward trend and the length of time between any rise. In most cases, the doubling of the PSA should be cause for concern, especially if it doubles in a short time. However, if you are 60 years old and your original PSA was 2.0 ng/ml, and it takes five years for it to double to 4.0 ng/ml, you may not have to worry. If your PSA is 10 ng/ml or less maybe you should have a free-to-total PSA. If the free percentage is above 20%, then you probably do not have to worry. You may not even need to have a biopsy.

But if you are 60 years old and your beginning PSA or base PSA (bPSA) is 2.0 ng/ml and a year later it is 4.0 ng/ml, then you would have to be concerned. If the free PSA is less than 20%, then a biopsy probably should be done. But remember that the first rule when it comes to cancer is that there are no rules. We are all different and most cancers are as different as we are. So we have no absolute way to determine which cancers are just pussy cats and which are tigers.

Prostate cancer is not the only problem many men have. If you are at least 70 years old, there is a 70% chance that you have Benign Prostatic Hyperplasia or BPH. If you are 80 years old the chances of having BPH is 80% and 100% if you are 100 years old. Not many men die because of BPH, but it can severely disrupt one's Quality of Life. There are several drugs and treatments for this disease. Sometimes a man with BPH can just Watch and Wait.

You should also know that if you are 80 years old, you probably have some prostate cancer along with the BPH. But it may not cause any problems.

So, if you have been diagnosed with prostate cancer, depending on your age, your health, expected life span, your PSA and your Gleason score, you may choose to just "Watch and Wait" (WW).However, Watch and Wait does not mean that you should do nothing about your prostate cancer. W.J. Kenney, a man who appreciates humor, said that he came across this line on the Internet regarding watchful waiting: "Ignoring prostate cancer is like trying to maintain eye contact while talking to Dolly Parton." Dr. Gerald Chodak, an advocate of this therapy, says that it should be called "Expectant Therapy". Others call it Watchful Progression. You should be aware that the natural history of prostate cancer is progression.

For some, it may take a long time and they may die with their prostate cancer, not from it. Or they may get run over by a truck or die of some other cause before the cancer kills them. But left unchecked, it will progress. In some cancers that progression can be very slow and may take a long time. It may never cause a problem. Other prostate cancers may grow very fast and be very aggressive. Again, the first rule when it comes to cancer is that there are no rules.

You should expect that eventually you will have to take some action. You should keep a close check on your PSA and any other signs of cancer activity, and be prepared to take appropriate action. We have several tools that allow us to keep a wary eye on the cancer for any sign of undue activity. We can then treat it accordingly. Our technology, tools and methods of diagnosis continue to improve.

There will come a day when we will be able to positively predict which tumors are the bad guys right from the beginning.

WHO SHOULD ADOPT WW?

Dr. Israel Barken and Ralph Valle make frequent posts to the Internet Prostate Problems Mailing List (PPML). (Instructions on how to join this list are given later in this chapter.)

Below are a couple of notes they posted to the PPML.

From Dr. Barken:

> <Many in the medical establishment feel that a patient may adopt WW if one or more of these four points are fulfilled:
>
> 1. Age above 70; 2. Significant medical problems; 3. Low volume and low grade tumor; 4. Diploid tumor. These points are the conclusion of an article reviewing 8 studies of watchful waiting. My personal view is that no patient has to fit perfectly to the rules. The key is for the patient to feel comfortable with what he is doing. Quality of life may be more important to patients than statistical likelihood of surviving a certain number of years. Watchful Waiting is a bad term. Watchful Doing is a much better term. Patients can do a lot before submitting to any primary treatment—Good nutrition, good exercise and good mental attitude are very important. Whatever he does, the patient has to feel comfortable while monitoring his situation.Take care, Israel Barken, MD>

Ralph Valle replied:

> <So true, people should be able to be comfortable with monitoring, but sadly, so many who could fit the mold of WW, get scared when they get the news, and too many doctors don't suggest, or explain, WW as a potential methodology when they fit the profile you mentioned.

> We have seen many posts by men who have gone
> through so much that suggests regret because of
> precipitous action. Those of us who have been on the
> PPML for several months are aware that many men are in
> fact doing something other than just sitting and waiting
> and watching the cancer cells multiply. Some are
> changing their life styles, changing to low-fat diets,
> eating soy products, taking saw palmetto, adopting high
> fiber diets, taking antioxidants, engaging in exercise,
> meditation, stress reduction, etc. Ralph>

There are several men who are ideal candidates for WW. None of us like to think about the end, but eventually it will come to all of us. Trying to predict how much time we have left is no fun but it should be part of any treatment decision. If you are 80 years old, you probably won't live another 25 years. But it is quite possible that you will live another 10 years. If you are diagnosed with prostate cancer, you probably should not consider having a radical prostatectomy. But we are all different. A member of a local support group had a radical prostatectomy at age 83. He expects to live for another 20 years. For most men at this age the major surgery may be quite traumatic. If you are an older person, you may die from some other disease before the prostate cancer kills you.

On the other hand, if you are 50 years old, normally you should expect to live for another 25 to 30 years. However, depending on your diagnostic stage, your PSA, your Gleason Score and your general health, your cancer could kill you within two to ten years. But if you are a 50 year old man, with a low PSA, a low Gleason Score, and otherwise in good health, then you may be a good candidate for watchful waiting.

Some of the advantages of watchful waiting include its initial freedom from side effects of harsh treatments. It may also be inexpensive since you will not be paying for drugs and treatments.

Watchful waiting may be best for those who are too old or too ill to withstand the rigors of treatment. It may be difficult to face reality, but if a man's life expectancy is fairly short, a radical treatment may not be worthwhile.

DON'T RUSH TO TREATMENT

There is no need to panic if you have just been diagnosed. It may have taken 10 or more years for your cancer to have become significant enough to be detected. It won't hurt to wait just a while longer. Before making a decision for any treatment, whether watchful waiting, surgery, radiation or any other modality, learn all you can about your disease first. Remember that your doctor may be very busy and may not have time to study your charts and tests. You should get copies of all your tests and records. Don't be put off if the doctor or hospital refuses to give them to you. Your records belong to you. You should study them. Always remember that it is your body, your disease, your life and your decision as to which treatments to choose.

GRAPH YOUR TRENDS

A very important tool is to make sure that you have several PSA readings so that you can look for a trend. Many men use graph paper to plot the activity of their PSA. The PSA will correlate fairly closely to the activity of the cancer. Some men use their computer and a spreadsheet program such as Lotus, Quattro or Excel to plot their PSA and other tests. All doctors and hospitals should use this type of record keeping. Most doctors have to wade through a large manila folder full of the patient's history and visit records. A spreadsheet program could show the doctor all of your tests, drugs and trends immediately. Eventually, this will happen.

John Fistere is a computer programming whiz. He has written a program called MultiGraph that will construct a graph for you showing the trends of your disease. All you have to do is send him a digest of your history by e-mail. It's a free service of the Prostate Cancer Research and Education Foundation (PCREF). Send a message to John at JFistere@email.msn.com for instructions. John has contributed a whole lot to the fight against prostate cancer.

John is a part-time Executive Director for PCREF.

6699 Alvarado Road
San Diego, CA 92120
Tel: 619-287-8866
Fax: 619-287-8890

The PSA will reflect to a great extent your cancer activity and should be monitored closely. This doesn't mean that you should be getting a PSA test every other day. Dr. E. David Crawford says that some men become "PSA junkies" who may shop around and get several PSAs, hoping to find a lab that returns a test that suits them. Depending on your diagnosis, stage, Gleason and other factors, you may not need a PSA more often than once every six months. Of course if it appears that your PSA is rising fast, then it should be done more often.

You should know your clinical stage and your Gleason score and know their significance. Knowing these numbers, you should consult the Partin and Narayan Tables in Chapter Six and determine the predictions.

LEARNING WHAT YOU NEED TO KNOW

Before you can make a good decision about any treatment you must be informed. We are talking about your life and how much longer you may live. How much longer you live may depend on the decisions you make. There are several good books on prostate cancer. Read them and learn. If you have a computer, log onto the various web sites and learn. A couple of the better sites are the Prostate Problems Help List (PHML) and the Prostate Problems Mailing List (PPML). These sites are actually e-mail sites. There are several hundred patients and relatives who post questions, problems and answers on these lists every day. A great many of the posts are from individuals who have had all of the various treatments. Their firsthand experiences can help you enormously. If you are going to have a treatment, what better way to find out what to expect than from someone who has had that treatment? Several doctors monitor the PHML and the PPML and answer questions. They usually point out that their answers and advice cannot take the place of a face-to-face consultation with your doctor. The subscriptions to PHML and PPML are free. All you need is a computer and a modem.

Of course you will need to access the PHML and PPML through an Internet Service Provider (ISP) such as AOL, Prodigy, Compuserve, or any of the hundreds of providers now available. The ISP services may cost about $20 or more per month. Many have local access telephone numbers, otherwise you may have to pay a telephone toll for time spent on the internet. To subscribe to the PPML and PHML use your E-Mail that is usually supplied by your IPS. When you log on to send a message a form will usually come up with space for address, subject and message. Send e-mail to:

    listserv@listserv.acor.org

    Subject—leave blank or put a dash if your software requires it.

    Message—subscribe Prostate firstname lastname

To subscribe to Prostate Help Mailing List or PHML send e-mail to:

    listserv@home.ease.lsoft.com

    subject: leave blank

    message: subscribe prostate help

You will be notified in a few hours to confirm that you wish to subscribe.

Another excellent web site is www.prostatepointers.org. Once you get to this site, you will see several places of interest. If you click on Medicine, you will find several articles about prostate cancer. The ProstatePointersweb site is maintained by Professor Gary Huckabay, a young man with advanced prostate cancer. He puts in many long hours maintaining the web site. He is also very active in the National Prostate Cancer Coalition (NPCC). If you don't have a computer, you should think about getting one. At one time, computers were very expensive but most everyone can afford them now.

SOME DISADVANTAGES OF WATCH AND WAIT

There are thousands of men who are doing very well on watch and wait. We don't want to frighten you, but there are some downsides to watch and wait. One problem is that some men may become complacent and not worry about their disease. They may have a false sense of security because they feel good. They may forget that prostate cancer usually has no early symptoms. They may also wait too long before seeking treatment. There is usually a window of opportunity when curative treatment can be initiated. Once the cancer has escaped the prostate, it is incurable. However, it is still treatable.

Another disadvantage is that we can only know the clinical stage of the cancer, which may not be the true stage. The patient may think he has an indolent cancer when in fact it may be a fairly dangerous beast. The patient may have read or heard of some of the Swedish and other studies that seem to prove that prostate cancer is something that needs no treatment. Many magazines and newspapers reported the studies with large headlines. Many people were led to believe that prostate cancer can be ignored. Many of the studies have been proven to have been flawed, but there have been no headlines and few magazine stories to refute the original reports.

WAITING TOO LONG

One of the early advocates of watchful waiting was Dr. Willet F. Whitmore of the Memorial Sloan-Kettering Cancer Center. He was one of the pioneers in brachytherapy. This was before we had ultrasound so they made an incision then placed the radioactive seeds by hand. They were not too successful.

Dr. Whitmore and Dr. Jewett developed the A B C D staging system for prostate cancer. Dr. Whitmore coined the phrase "Is cure necessary for those in whom it is possible and is cure possible in those for whom it is necessary?"

Here is another quote from Dr. Whitmore:

"Many more men die with prostate cancer than of it. Growing old is invariably fatal. Prostate cancer is only sometimes so."

Dr. Whitmore was stricken with prostate cancer himself. He chose to watch and wait. He later died of prostate cancer. Shortly before he died, it was reported that he said he regretted the fact that he had waited too long before actively treating his disease.

There is definitely a window of opportunity for cure. We have several tools that can help recognize that window. But none of them are absolute.

CONSERVATIVE TREATMENTS

With some radical treatments there is a diminishing of quality of life. But newer treatments, procedures and technologies are being developed such as cryosurgery and various types of radiation such as 3D Conformal External Beam radiation, Proton Beam radiation and seed implants. These newer treatments can save your life and may have very little effect on diminishing your quality of life. Even if a treatment diminishes your quality of life, it is still better than not being alive.

There are some studies ongoing that are using high dose antiandrogens as a chemoprevention and treatment. Theoretically, the antiandrogens such as Flutamide, Casodex or Nilutamide are synthetic drugs that appear to the cancer cells to be real androgens. These drugs can attach to the androgen receptors of the cancer cells, then when the real androgen comes along, the cell is already satisfied. The real androgen is thus blocked. Without the real androgens, the cell will starve and die. The cells also need testosterone in the form of dihydrotestosterone (DHT). An enzyme, 5alpha-reductase, is needed to convert testosterone to DHT. Proscar is an inhibitor of 5alpha-reductase. The prostate cancer cells must have the DHT in order to survive.

Some men are taking 150mg/day of casodex and 5mg of proscar. We don't have any long-term data, but most seem to be doing well. The high dose antiandrogens have very few side effects. However breast enlargement or gynecomastia is almost universal. Many men have a small dose of radiation to their breasts which prevents the enlargement.

One large disadvantage of the LHRH agonists such as Lupron or Zoladex is that these drugs eliminate the production of testosterone. Without testosterone, there is no libido. Without testosterone, there is also loss of muscle mass, fatigue and osteoporosis or bone loss. The high dose casodex or flutamide does not affect the production of testosterone, but they help prevent it from being utilized by the cancer cells.

If you can determine that your prostate cancer is slow growing, you can easily monitor it. New methods of treatment are being developed every day. New research is very promising. If you can hold off long enough, perhaps the "magic bullet" will be discovered before you have to have a radical treatment.

CHEMOPREVENTION

For the last 11 years, co-author Dr. E. David Crawford has organized an International Prostate Cancer Update Conference. A special addition to one of his Conferences addressed the Progress and Prospects for Chemoprevention of Prostate Cancer. He had several renowned speakers such as Drs. Fernand Labrie, David Bostwick, Charles Boone, Brian Henderson, Gary Kelloff and several others. Their presented data shows that prostate cancer can be avoided in many cases. One of the better treatments of all is to prevent prostate cancer. Chemoprevention of prostate cancer means using drugs such as the antiandrogens, antioxidants, use of vitamins and minerals, diet, exercise and good common sense health practices.

We haven't found the magic bullet yet, but we are getting closer.

Chapter Eight
RADICAL PROSTATECTOMY
By Dr. E. David Crawford

Cancer of the prostate may be cured when it remains contained within the prostate and may respond to therapy even when widespread; survival is intimately linked with the extent of the tumor. Controversy continues to exist regarding the appropriate treatment of patients with prostate cancer, especially in the early stages. This is partly due to the variable history of the disease and also the inability to predict individual outcomes. In addition to the extent of the tumor, other factors such as patient age and state of health, influence treatment choices. Several options are available for cancer that has not yet escaped the prostate including surgery, different types of radiation and cryosurgery.

Some people may be a bit confused when they first hear the term radical prostatectomy. If you look in the dictionary, you will find several different definitions and adjectives to describe radical such as extreme, drastic, fanatical, revolutionary, freak, maniac, and many others. But in medical terminology, radical means a treatment that seeks an absolute cure.

Radical treatments are usually the opposites of palliative or conservative treatments. A palliative treatment is something used to ease or give temporary relief without curing. A simple prostatectomy may be done on a patient with BPH where only the inner portions of the prostatic urethra may be removed. (See Chapter Five). When a radical prostatectomy is done, the entire prostate and seminal vesicles are removed.

Radical prostatectomies have been performed for more than 100 years. The two main methods used in removing the prostate and its associated structures are the perineal and retropubic approach.

SURGERY

Until just a few years ago, our treatment choices were limited to surgery or external radiation. We now have other choices including "watchful waiting" which is based on the premise the cancer may be slowly progressive, radioactive seed implants, and cryosurgery which freezes the prostate killing the malignant cells. Radical prostate surgery, however, is still the "gold standard" for localized prostate cancer. If detected in time, it is the only treatment that can completely remove the cancer, providing it is entirely contained within the prostate capsule.

A radical prostatectomy is a major surgery and may not be the treatment of choice for all patients. Very few doctors would perform such an operation on an 80-year-old man because the trauma of the surgery might cause him more harm than the cancer. Some physicians will not even consider a 75-year-old man a good candidate for surgery. We are all different; there are some 75-year-old men who will live another 20 years while others will die within the next few months.

The various other forms of therapies and treatments may fail to eradicate all of the cancer cells. However, in some cases, it may take several years for any of these cancer cells to become significant. So these treatments may be okay for an older man with a fairly short life expectancy or one who may not be able to withstand the trauma of the major surgery. He might die of other causes before the cancer could kill him.

Because it holds the promise of removing all cancer cells, a radical prostatectomy may be the treatment of choice for a younger man in his 40s or 50s with a long life expectancy. A big problem is that we have no way of knowing for sure whether the cancer is still totally confined to the prostatic capsule. Despite our best clinical tests, about 10% to 20% of the prostate cancers believed to be local have already established micrometastases somewhere else in the body. This means the cancer may recur within the next five to ten years in one of every five men who have a radical prostatectomy.

THE RADICAL RETROPUBIC PROSTATECTOMY

Dr. T. Millin pioneered the radical retropubic prostatectomy (RRP) in 1947. (The prostate lies behind the pubic bone and below the bladder; the word retropubic means behind the pubic bone). Over the years, the group at Johns Hopkins have greatly refined the prostatectomy procedure. They discovered the fact that nerves and blood vessels that control erections lie alongside the prostate. Until the 1980s, these nerves and blood vessels were automatically removed during a prostatectomy. This meant the man would never again be able to have a normal erection. Surgical techniques have been developed that can spare the nerves and blood vessels so the man can still maintain his potency.

Until 1947, most prostatectomies were done through the perineum. The perineum is that area located between the scrotum and anus. Though the prostate is easier to access utilizing the perineal approach, it doesn't allow much room to work and limits the view of the gland. This procedure also does not allow the lymph nodes to be inspected and removed. The retropubic approach is now used in the majority of all radical prostatectomies performed today. This procedure provides a better view of the prostatic area and is less complicated than the perineal approach. It provides access to the lymph nodes, gives better control over bleeding and provides a more precise anatomic dissection of the prostate.

AUTOLOGOUS BLOOD DONATION

Patients are usually asked to make an autologous donation of two units of blood prior to their operation. (The prefix *auto* is Greek for self, *logos* is Greek for word or reason, meaning that something had its origin within an individual. If one needs a blood transfusion, a person's own blood is best).

In doing a retropubic procedure, an incision is made from the navel to the pubic bone. Large circular retractors are used to separate and hold the incision apart to provide a wide field of vision. There are lots of blood vessels in the pelvic area and having a wide field of vision makes it easier for the surgeon to identify and tie off pesky vessels. If the blood vessels are not properly tied off and the bleeding controlled, the patient could lose a very large amount of blood.

Most experienced doctors can do a prostatectomy with less than one unit. In our practice in Denver, using techniques we have developed, none of our last 250 patients have required a blood transfusion.

We have been using a new tool that saves us time and saves a loss of blood.

Figure 8-1 shows the LigaSure system. The scissor-like device is clamped onto a blood vessel. Electrical energy passes through the device and seals the blood vessel and severs it.

Ordinarily, the surgeon has to ligate or place a catgut string around each blood vessel in two places, then cut the vessel between the ligations. Ligating and tying off blood vessels can be time consuming and may also result in a loss of blood. The LigaSure system saves time and is more effective than ligation. The system is fairly new, but we expect that many surgeons will soon be using it.

THE PROSTATE AND BLADDER VALVE

The prostate is shaped somewhat like an upside down pyramid. Its base is attached to the primary bladder sphincter or the main urinary valve. The apex is attached to a set of muscles on the pelvic floor. Some of these muscles encircle the urethra and form a secondary sphincter or musculomembranous valve. Some doctors call the primary bladder sphincter the internal valve and the secondary valve, the external valve. If the main bladder valve is damaged, we are forced to rely on the secondary musculomembranous valve to control our bladder functions.

This secondary valve must be trained in order to take over the urinary voiding function. If the secondary valve was not damaged, this training can usually be accomplished by doing Kegel exercises. In a small number of cases, both valves may be damaged. In such a circumstance, the patient may have severe incontinence problems. Urinary incontinence following a prostatectomy is not always due to sphincter insufficiency but sometimes to bladder muscle dysfunction, or both. (More about Kegel exercises and incontinence in Chapter Seventeen.)

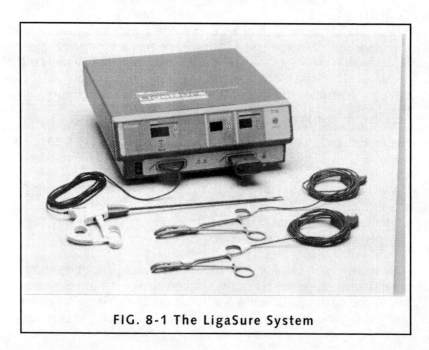

FIG. 8-1 The LigaSure System

THE FOLEY CATHETER

Before the operation begins, a Foley catheter is inserted through the penis into the bladder. The catheter is a rubber tube with an inflatable balloon on the end. Once the catheter is inserted into the bladder, using a syringe, the balloon is inflated with sterile water through a small tube that runs parallel to the main catheter; the inflated balloon keeps the catheter from falling out. During the operation, the catheter is used to help lift the prostate up so that it is easier to cut it out and remove it.

From apex to base, the prostate is about one inch long. During a prostatectomy, the prostate and the portion of the urethra within it are removed. When the prostate is cut away from the bladder, it leaves a hole about one inch in diameter. The base of the prostate and urethra is severed from the bladder. The apex is then severed from the pelvic musculo-membraneous tissues. The bladder is then pulled down and the severed end of the urethra is sewn to the bladder. The surgeon stitches the bladder in such a way, called a tennis racket procedure, so as to reduce the size of the bladder opening to fit the urethra.

This junction is called a urethral anastomosis. Occasionally, scar tissue from the anastomosis may cause voiding problems. The scar tissue can usually be reamed out successfully.

A second catheter, called a suprapubic catheter, is sometimes inserted into the bladder through a small abdominal incision. Both catheters are connected to drainage bags to collect the urine. The suprapubic catheter is removed after a few days, but the Foley catheter remains in place for 10 days to two weeks to allow time for the newly formed bladder neck to heal.

Depending on the artistry and skill of the surgeon, as well as patient selection, the patient may experience few, if any, problems with incontinence. Following the removal of the urinary catheter, adult diapers or pads may be required until control is regained. Usually, the incontinence is mild and generally requires only one to three pads per day. Most men can regain control and be completely dry within two to three weeks.

Though a substantial majority of men regain total urinary control over time, a few (5-15%) are left with severe incontinence and may require additional treatment. The primary bladder valve is intimately connected to the base of the prostate. This valve can be damaged during a radical prostatectomy. Mild urinary stress incontinence (involuntary loss of urine associated with physical exertion such as coughing or sneezing) may be experienced in up to 15-20% of patients after radical prostatectomy. Several studies involving the use of surgical techniques designed to conserve continence, while not compromising removal of the cancer, have demonstrated favorable outcomes.

The length of time for surgery varies from two to three hours, depending on the expertise of the surgeon and any unforeseen patient complications. Before you have surgery, make sure you find an experienced and highly skilled surgeon.

DR. CRAWFORD'S TECHNIQUE:

As has been discussed there are a number of ways to remove the prostate. An advantage in using my technique is that the gland is not penetrated before the blood vessels are ligated. Since the blood vessels are all tied off before cutting into the prostate, it may prevent the cancer cells from being spread into the system. This may help prevent metastasis. This is theoretical and not proven. The most significant advantage is that the dorsal vein complex which is the major source of blood loss during the procedure is the last step in the procedure. In over 1700 of these operations, I have never had a case of rectal injury. In the past 250 cases there has not been one patient who has required a blood transfusion.

Utilizing the LigaSure device has permitted us to develop a method to spare the bladder neck and thus leads to earlier control of urine. The device is used to seal the dorsal vein complex and arteries. We believe this provides better continence control since we don't have to place a lot of sutures in this area to control bleeding. Ordinarily, a lot bleeding in this area may necessitate the use of many sutures which could damage the continence mechanism.

The use of the CaverMap has helped to further improve the potency rate.

LYMPH NODES

It is frequently difficult to determine the exact stage of prostate cancer and quite often it is underestimated. Staging involves the gathering of information to determine, as precisely as possible, the exact extent of tumor spread, both at the site of origin, and in sites of metastasis. Staging is of critical importance since the best treatment plan for a patient is based on the stage of the disease. Staging is also essential to formulating a prognosis.

Cancer of the prostate may spread by direct extension, the blood stream, the nerves and the lymphatic system. The first site of local spread beyond the prostate is usually to the pelvic lymph nodes and often goes undetected. Studies from past years have shown that these structures will be positive for cancer cells in 5-50% of patients at the time they present with prostate cancer. The prognosis is worse in patients who have involvement of the pelvic lymph nodes. But we now use PSA extensively so most cancers are now detected earlier. Because of the earlier detection, the lymph node involvement is decreasing. This is another good reason for screening.

It is possible for metastasis to occur without pelvic lymph node involvement. Remember, however, the first rule about cancer is that there are no rules!

ARTIFICIAL NEURAL NETWORKS

Using computers, databases and networks, we have recently employed Artificial Neural Networks (ANNs) on our patients. The ANN seems to be very accurate in selecting those patients who may have lymph node disease. In general, if the PSA is less than ten and the Gleason score is less than 7, the probability of lymph node involvement is rather slight.

Here is an abstract about ANNs:

Artificial Intelligence System In Prediction Of Lymph Node Involvement In Radical Prostatectomy Patients

E David Crawford 1; Peter Snow 2; John Lynch 3; David McLeod 3; Joseph Batuello 1; Alan Partin 4; Richard Stock 5; Nelson Stone 5; Eduard Gamito 1; Jeffrey Brandt 2; 1 Denver, CO; 2 Colorado Springs, CO; 3 Washington, DC; 4 Baltimore, MD; 5 New York, NY (Presented by E David Crawford)

Objectives:

Approximately 125,000 radical prostatectomies are performed annually as treatment for prostate cancer in the US. Depending on the surgeon and institution, a pelvic lymphadenectomy is often performed as part of these procedures. Approximately 5-10% of patients that have lymphadenectomy with radical prostatectomy have pathology proven lymph node disease. Therefore, approximately 90-95% of these lymphadenectomies are unnecessary. An accurate method for identifying patients with a low risk for lymph node involvement would help eliminate unnecessary procedures and would provide a significant savings in morbidity and cost for patients and the health care system. An Artificial Intelligence (AI) system was employed to assign patients to a low risk group with high accuracy.

Methods:

An AI system consisting of a binary recursive partitioning technology and an artificial neural network was developed to assign patients to a low risk group. A database of 4,133 patient records was used to train and validate the AI system.

The three input variables studied were TNM stage, Gleason sum score and preoperative PSA. The output variable was lymph node involvement. After training and validation on this database, the same AI system was tested on a smaller database (227 records) from another institution. PSA and Gleason cut-off values derived by the AI system were also evaluated using the Partin Nomogram Tables.

Results:

The AI system was able to assign approximately 55% of the patients in the large database to a low risk group with an accuracy of 98-99% (1-2% false negatives). The AI system was able to assign approximately 25% of the patients in the smaller database to a low risk group with an accuracy of 98-99% (1-2% false negatives). PSA and Gleason cut-off values from the AI system of <10.35 ng/mL and 6, respectively, were applied to the Partin Tables and comparable results were achieved. The percentage of patients assigned to the low risk group varied between databases (25% and 55%).

Conclusion:

This AI system is the first in the field of predicting lymph node disease in prostate cancer to be trained and validated using data from one institution and then tested on data from another institution with consistent results. Using this technology, we can identify patients at low risk for lymph node involvement with an accuracy of 98-99% and thereby avoid performing unnecessary lymphadenectomies on these patients. The data suggest that between 25% to 55% of lymphadenectomies performed each year can be eliminated providing a significant potential cost savings. These results are consistent with those obtained using a variety of neural network architectures by other investigators and appear to be more dependent on the information contained in the clinical variables rather than a specific neural network. An increase in the number of input variables (3 were used in this study) as well as improving the quality of databases should increase the accuracy of AI systems in predicting nodal involvement in prostate cancer.

Source: 1999 AUA Meeting

LAPAROSCOPIC PELVIC LYMPH NODE DISSECTION

The only conclusive way of establishing nodal disease is by a biopsy. This biopsy may be done during a radical prostatectomy when the patient is first opened. The nearby lymph nodes are dissected, quick frozen and analyzed by a pathologist before the operation proceeds.

It may also be desirable to analyze the lymph nodes if radiation is conducted. When a retropubic approach is selected, the lymph nodes are readily accessible and easy to remove so they can be checked for cancer cells. If a radical perineal prostatectomy is done, an incision through the abdomen is required to access the nodes. Removal of the lymph nodes using a laparoscope (laparoscopic lymphadenectomy) can usually be accomplished with fewer patient complications than removal of the nodes through a separate abdominal approach. The laparoscope is a small instrument that can be inserted into the pelvic region through a small incision in the abdomen. It may have a camera and lens arrangement that can be attached to a television monitor.

The laparascope allows visualization and may also be fitted with cutting blades and retrieval forceps to remove lymph nodes. A laparoscopic lymphadenectomy avoids an abdominal incision and pelvic drains. It may also cause minimal postoperative discomfort and a shorter hospital stay.

It may not be necessary to do a pelvic lymph node examination in some cases. As reported in the October 1995 Journal of Urology, Dr. Nelson Stone and others performed laparoscopic studies on 157 patients. PSA scores of 4 or less were not associated with metastases. In addition, metastases were not identified with a Gleason score of 4 or less. The group found no metastases affiliated with most clinical stages T1a, b, or c. Several lymph nodes were positive for cancer when the PSA levels were greater than 4.1, Gleason scores above 5, and clinical stage T2 or more. The authors reported a 48% chance of finding positive nodes and seminal vesicle invasion with a Gleason score of 7 and above and a PSA value greater than 20 ng/ml.

TO PROCEED OR NOT

Like many aspects of prostate cancer and treatments, there can be controversy as to how to proceed if the lymph nodes are positive. In doing a retropubic operation, the lymph nodes are readily accessible. If it appears that the patient is at risk, the nodes are removed and sent to the pathology lab, quick frozen and checked for cancer. If the nodes are found to be positive for cancer cells, the operation may be halted without removing the prostate.

Many doctors believe the trauma of having a major operation, and the risk of incontinence and impotence, are not worth any perceived benefits. There is an old saying, "It does no good to lock the barn door after the horse has escaped."

However, there are some doctors who feel that removing the main source of the tumor helps to significantly reduce the tumor burden and is thus beneficial. A large cooperative study indicated that there is a survival advantage to removing the prostate and beginning immediate hormonal therapy.

EXTRACAPSULAR EXTENSION AND POSITIVE MARGINS

Usually, there is not much extra tissue surrounding the prostate, especially between the peripheral zone and the rectum. The surgeon, while taking out the prostate and associated structures, will attempt to remove as much fat and extra tissue as possible. In this way, any cancer cells existing outside the prostatic capsule may be removed as well. The excised tissues surrounding the prostate are called the margins. The surgically detached prostate, seminal vesicles, and extra tissue margins are referred to as the specimen.

All indications may be that the tumor is completely encapsulated. However, when the specimen is examined, the pathologist may find the prostatic capsule penetrated, or medically speaking, the presence of extracapsular extension (ECE). The pathologist will also inspect the margins for cancer cells, and if found, the margins are said to be surgically positive. If cancer cells cannot be detected, the margins are referred to as surgically negative. Negative margins usually indicate confinement of the cancer to the prostate, whereas, positive margins signify local spread, at the very least.

Cancers confined within the prostatic capsule rarely recur, having a local recurrence rate of approximately 2% and a distant recurrence rate of 1%. Patients with positive margins are at increased risk for local and distant cancer recurrence and about 50% will have a recurrence.

If the cancer has spread into the seminal vesicles or other pelvic structures, surgical removal of all cancer cells may not be possible. In this case, quite often the patient will undergo a series of external beam radiation treatments (XRT). A few doctors will also treat the patient with hormone therapy such as Lupron plus Flutamide or Casodex or Zoladex plus Flutamide or Casodex.

The PSA will also be closely monitored. Changes in the PSA level are reflective of changes in disease activity. PSA levels detectable after radical prostatectomy usually indicate local treatment failure or metastatic disease.

CLINICAL STAGE VS. PATHOLOGICAL STAGE

Prior to the time the prostate is removed and sent to the pathologist for a histological or microscopic examination, the diagnosis is just a clinical estimate of the stage of the disease. Even the biopsy Gleason grade may not be true because some of the cancer may have been missed.

After the prostate is removed, the pathologist can look at slices of the prostate and determine the true Gleason grade and make a more accurate estimate of the stage of disease. Tissues are graded according to their ability to retain their normal appearance. The more disrupted the normal glandular architecture, the higher the grade of tumor and the poorer the prognosis.

If the pathologist finds cancer cells have penetrated the capsule, or extracapsular extension, the stage is at least a C or T3a. A pathologic stage is indicated by placing a "p" before the stage. For example, a clinical stage C2 would be indicated as pathological stage pC2 or pT3.

NERVE SPARING

Until 1982, when a radical prostatectomy was performed, the prostate and all of the adjacent nerves and blood vessels were routinely removed. Until the early 1980s, most radical prostatectomies were done by the perineal approach. Following surgery, almost all of the patients were left permanently impotent which caused some patients to shun the procedure.

Investigators set about identifying the nerves and blood vessels that innervate the corpora cavernosa of the penis. The corpora cavernosa are two cylindrical masses of erectile tissue located on each side of the penis. When this tissue becomes engorged with arterial blood, an erection is created. The nerves and blood vessels, or neurovascular bundle, responsible for erections are attached to each side of the prostate. A procedure was developed whereby the neurovascular bundle could be identified, gently stripped away and "spared." Most urologists refer to this type of prostatectomy as "nerve sparing."

Nerve sparing may also play a minor role in the recovery of urinary control.

CAVERMAP

The erectile nerves may be very difficult to detect. We are all different so the location of the neurovascular bundle may be different from man to man. Unless the surgeon is very careful, the neurovascular bundle can be damaged or severed.

The Bard Uromed Company has developed an instrument that can be used to locate and identify the neurovascular bundle. A strain gauge ring is placed around the base of the patient's penis. This ring can detect minute responses to nerve stimulation to the penis which causes an engorgement. This ring is connected to the electronic instrument. A probe that is connected to the instrument is used to explore the areas on the sides of the exposed prostate.

When a nerve is contacted, it sends a signal through the nerve which is detected by the ring on the base of the penis. As a result of the erection a signal is sent to the instrument for visual verification.

After the operation is complete, the probe can again be placed against the nerve and if the nerve is still intact, it will send a signal to the ring on the base of the penis.

Here is some information from the Uromed web site at www.uromed.com :

"The CaverMap surgical aid is a combination nerve stimulator and erectile response detection system for intraoperative use during surgery. The system generates a stimulation current which is emitted from several electrodes on the probe tip. The probe tip is placed on tissue that is suspect of containing sensitive nerves or significant nerve branches. When the physician stimulates this tissue, the device detects erectile responses in the form of minute changes in penile circumference. Based on the presence or absence of a confirmed response, physicians can make informed decisions regarding the dissection pattern to be used for the particular anatomy in each patient.

Rapid determination of nerve function: response cycle as fast as 20 seconds. Confirms status of nerve function intraoperatively.

Reaches difficult areas: flexible probe tip and ergonomic handle offer 180 degree range.

Audible and visible tumescence response: light and sound indicators.

Detects nerve presence through penile tumescence changes: ultra-sensitive tumescence strain gauge. (The ring at the base of the penis.)

Broad to narrow field of nerve stimulation: 8 individually controlled electrodes on probe tip in a range from 0.2 to 1.0 cm wide."

NERVE GRAFTS

A few doctors are now doing nerve grafts when the erectile nerves must be removed. They remove a short piece of a nerve in the ankle area of the foot and connect it between the severed ends of the nerves. The nerve graft must be done at the same time that the prostate is removed.

For more information about this new experimental technique being performed at The Methodist Hospital please call (713) 790-

3333 or submit your questions through the <u>Ask the Doctor </u>section of our website.

http://methodisthealth.com/SCOOP/graft.htm

Here is a post to the internet from a man who had the sural nerve graft:

> Subj: My success after sural nerve graft
>
> From: BoyettC@aol.com
>
> Hi all,
>
> My RRP with one sural nerve graft was 3-24-99. I am unable to take Viagra because of heart medication. I have tried a VED and I should use it more. My ED specialist and also urologist, wants me to use it 15 minutes daily. It had slipped his mind that I couldn't take Viagra and until I reminded him he wanted me to use Viagra also along with the VED. He also suggested trying the Trimix injections but I decided to hold off on that for the time being. But now wish I had gone ahead and let him give me the prescription and instruct me on it's use.
>
> Just since the middle of August and before getting the VED, I have had a little response with lots of mental and manual stimulation. I emphasize the little. But I was really glad to get a response and it gives me hope for the future. Of course since we had one nerve graft with the other spared we will never know which or if both nerves are working. And of course don't care as long as we get the desired response.
>
> My foot especially around the ankle area remains numb on the outside and when touching that area it feels "dead". But there are feelings under the skin and around the part of the ankle that wasn't involved with the incision. At the other incision, at the lower back of the leg, it feels almost normal now.
>
> My understanding is that the numbness will continue indefinitely and that doesn't relate to whether or not the grafted nerve produces erectile function. It doesn't really bother me any longer. I believe where the nerve was harvested, the cut nerve ends are "buried" into muscle. In the original graft study, or either in information provided prior to surgery, I remember at first they were not "buried" into the muscle and that caused more problems with nerve sensations or pain.
>
> The original nerve graft study by Dr. Scardino, Dr. Kim (my ED specialist) and Dr. Nath (the nerve surgeon) and others goes into quite a bit of detail.
>
> If you want to read it go to: http://www.urol.bcm.tmc.edu/wwwroot/GRAFT.html

Unfortunately for many men, the nerve graft must be done at the time of the prostatectomy. It is too early to know the ultimate success of this procedure.

One doctor who participated in a nerve graft operation complained that the services of the plastic surgeon were very expensive. The plastic surgeon who did the removal of the nerve and the microsurgery was paid more than the doctors who did the major operation.

WHY THE NERVES MAY NOT BE SAVED

Both before and during the time of surgery, the doctor tries to determine if the cancer has escaped the prostatic capsule. If the cancer has perforated it, there is a danger that it is in the nerves and blood vessels. If the cancer has escaped the capsule, the surgeon will not try to preserve the neurovascular bundle. It is possible the cancer will only be on one side of the prostate and invaded the neurovascular bundle on that side only. In this situation, the doctor can spare the nerves on the one good side.

If the patient was potent before the operation, he should still be able to have an erection postoperatively, although time to recovery of erections may take longer.

In some cases, even if both nerves are spared, some men will be impotent. This is true especially for many older patients. Age is a critical factor and it could be a multifactorial problem not yet fully understood. Some studies indicate that potency can be preserved in 91% of men younger than 50; 75% in men age 50-60; and 25% in men over the age of 70. This data applied to men who had both neurovascular bundles left intact. If one of the bundles had to be removed, the above figures were reduced by half.

Many fear surgery and most of the other treatments. You should keep in mind that the natural history of prostate cancer is progression. So even if there is a chance that you will be completely impotent, depending on the stage of cancer, an operation may prolong your life. If the cancer is detected early, there is a very good chance that you will still live a fairly long life. You can use several alternatives to still have a fairly good sex life.

RADICAL PERINEAL PROSTATECTOMY

The perineum is that area between the scrotum and anus. According to Dr. David Paulson, writing in Campbell's Urology, the perineal approach has been used for over 2000 years to reach the prostate and bladder. A radical perineal prostatectomy was first performed by Kuchier in 1866, soon after the availability of anesthesia. It wasn't until 1904, however, that it became popularized.

The radical retropubic prostatectomy and pelvic lymph node dissection, utilizing an abdominal approach, replaced the radical perineal prostatectomy when it was realized that unrecognized lymph node metastases was one of the causes of disease progression in many patients. Because this approach affords easy access to the lymph nodes, provides a better view of the prostatic area and allows for more precise anatomic dissection of the prostate, it has become the most widely used method today.

Radical perineal prostatectomy for cancer involves the removal of the entire gland, its capsule and seminal vesicles through the perineum. During surgery, the patient remains in a lithotomy position similar to a woman having a gynecological exam. The patient's legs are placed in stirrups and the penis and testicles are moved up and out of the operative area. The surgeon makes a crosswise incision, similar to the smile on a happy face drawing, between the scrotum and the anus. The prostate is then removed through this incision.

The literature indicates a higher incidence of incontinence, impotence and rectal injuries using the perineal approach. Some doctors believe the perineal approach to be inferior to the retropubic method. Drs. Joseph Mokulis and Ian Thompson disagree. Reporting in the January 1997 issue of the Journal of Urology, they claim it is much easier to use the perineal approach. They report using less blood (sometimes none at all), shorter operative times, and decreased patient hospital time. They also feel it takes less time for the patient to heal. They utilize this approach in selected patients and claim that it is a safe and effective operation when performed by a surgeon well trained in this surgery.

At the Fifth Annual International Conference (1995) on prostate cancer, it was suggested that radical perineal prostatectomy has once again found favor among some urologists. Based on reports, pelvic lymph node dissection may not be necessary in as many as 60-70% of patients with a less than 4% risk of positive nodes. If it appears necessary, a laparoscopic lymph node examination can be done before the surgery. Most patients selected for the perineal approach are those with organ confined disease (OCD). They may have low PSAs and Gleason Scores so there may be little need to sample the lymph nodes.

Postoperative pain may be dramatically reduced, complications reduced and the number of transfusions minimized using the perineal approach. There is less patient discomfort, more rapid return of appetite and bowel function and a lessened length of hospital stay. At one time it was standard practice to keep the patient in the hospital for about a week after a radical retropubic or perineal prostatectomy. Because of the high cost of hospitalization, many patients are now discharged after only 2 days.

A suggestion was made that cancer control and preservation of physiologic function can be achieved in properly selected patients to a degree comparable to radical retropubic prostatectomy. Laparoscopic pelvic lymph node dissection combined with radical perineal prostatectomy is considered an alternative to radical retropubic prostatectomy and lymph node removal.

RADICAL LAPAROSCOPIC PROSTATECTOMY

Dr. Crawford had a movie of the laparascopic RP at his 10th International PCa Update. A French and a German team are doing them in Europe. They use specialized instruments that must fit through the tubular laparoscopes. The laparoscope may be about 1/2 inch in diameter. It takes a lot of training to be able to manipulate the instruments through the laparoscopes and to cut, tie and to remove the tissue.

One or more of the laparoscopes have a light and another one or two is used to force carbon dioxide gas into the abdomen to open it up. One or more laparoscopes are equipped with a small camera which is hooked into a TV. So all of the work is done by watching the TV.

This procedure requires from 4 to 6 hours to perform it. An experienced urologist can do a RP in about 2 hours.

Other than the smaller scars, I cannot see any possible advantage for using a procedure such as this.

RECURRENCE

Despite the fact that a radical prostatectomy, the "gold standard," is the most effective way to remove the cancer, it is not perfect. In about 20% of the time, the cancer will recur within five years. This means that eithera few cells were left in the prostatic bed within the pelvic region, or some cells had already escaped and set up micro colonies before the surgery. We are constantly searching for new markers, tests and treatments that can improve our rate of success.

One of the best ways to beat cancer is early detection. Every incurable metastatic cancer was at one time a small localized cancer that could have been cured. **The answer to cancer is early detection!**

ULTRASENSITIVE PSA

After surgery, a significant number of patients may remain symptom free for extended periods of time. But any rise in the PSA after a prostatectomy should be cause for concern. The standard PSA test usually measures down to 0.2 ng/ml which is considered undetectable. Before treatment, there can be quite a lot of variation in the bPSA or beginning PSA. But after a prostatectomy, there should be no PSA at all by standard PSA tests. If there is, it means that somewhere in your body, prostate cancer cells are making PSA.

As with all cancer, the sooner you can find out about such cells, before they become too numerous, the easier it is to control them. The standard PSA test may not detect a small rise but there are several companies who now do ultrasensitive PSA tests.

Before treatment an ultrasensitive PSA test would not be necessary because of the wide variability of the PSA. The post treatment tests, especially after a prostatectomy, should be no greater than 0.2 with the standard test. If you suspect that your post treatment PSA is rising, you might want to have an ultrasensitive test done. It is imperative that you monitor your post treatment PSA. An ultrasensitive test can let you know very early if the PSA is rising. This would allow one to start early treatment before the cancer has a chance to gain a foothold.

SALVAGE TREATMENTS FOR FAILED THERAPIES

None of our therapies can guarantee a cure. In reality, many of the treatments fail at some time. But there are several treatment options for failures. Many of them do offer extended survival.

Rising PSA after a local therapy such as radical prostatectomy, radiation therapy, or seed implants signals a failure. In the past, the only way we would know that a man failed therapy would be the symptoms that appeared from spread of the disease. Now, we have a simple blood test that can give us a lead time of many years before there is a problem. A rise in PSA after local therapy gives us the opportunity to choose a number of different approaches, including just watching the PSA level.

PSA has been called the most important tumor marker in oncology. Certainly in prostate cancer, it has revolutionized our ability to detect the disease early, as well as follow the course of the disease in patients after being treated with different therapies. Following a successful radical prostatectomy, all prostate tissue should be removed and the PSA should be undetectable. Some assays report a level of 0, while others report less than .2 ng/ml. If the PSA level begins to elevate after a radical prostatectomy, this usually signals failure of treatment. However, it does not mean the patient is going to succumb to prostate cancer.

Once it is established that the PSA is rising, it is usually advisable to search for disease beyond the prostate. This may include a bone scan and, under some circumstances, a ProstaScint scan. This radionuclide scan is a monoclonal antibody directed to prostate specific membrane antigen (PSMA). Unlike PSA, PSMA is more frequently expressed in aggressive cancers. In one study of 180 men with rising PSAs, 60% showed a positive scan, 34% of those were positive in the area where the prostate was removed. This suggested a local recurrence. Prostate scan has a 49% sensitivity and a 71% specificity.

With these tests, the physician tries to determine whether the cancer represents a local recurrence, a distant event (usually in bone or lymph nodes), or a combination of both.

In some cases, a biopsy of the prostate or the prostatic bed is performed following either radiation or radical prostatectomy. Unfortunately, none of these tests provide 100% assurance that we are only dealing with a local recurrence. For example, a patient may have a PSA that has gone from 0 to .5 ng/ml to 1.0 ng/ml, years after a radical prostatectomy. A bone scan and ProstaScint scan may be negative, but unrecognized disease could still exist in distant places. Nevertheless, if a bone scan is positive for disease that is usually strong evidence that disease is beyond the prostate.

If a biopsy or a ProstaScint test indicates that the cancer is still in the prostatic bed, then radiation may be used. The patient may also be treated with hormone therapy.

Even though prostate cancer is detected early and the prostatectomy specimen shows a cancer confined to the prostate, failure can still occur. Not everyone who has a cancer that falls within the above criteria is cured. Somewhere between 5%-20% of these patients will eventually fail. We don't always know why it happens, but some possibilities include a local recurrence possibly from prostate tissue left behind, implantation of cancer into the area of removal which occurred at the time of surgery, or possibly unrecognized early spread of the disease even when it was confined to the prostate.

Salvage prostatectomy offers a chance to cure some patients who fail radiation therapy. The keys to selecting these patients are by evaluating the stage and grade of the cancer, their longevity, their quality of life concerns, and overall health. We have performed a number of these procedures and actually do it from a perineal approach beneath the scrotum. The procedure is well-tolerated, and most patients are only hospitalized 24 hours. Unfortunately, the majority of patients who undergo this procedure who were potent before, are impotent afterwards. This is due to the fact that there is an extensive amount of reaction around the prostate and it is difficult to do a nerve-sparing procedure after radiation therapy. There is also a risk of incontinence—and even in patients who are ultimately not incontinent, it takes months before control of the urine returns.

Even though there are no studies that suggest hormonal therapy will improve survival, there are some suggestions that early hormonal therapy is better than later. We believe that there is a survival advantage with hormonal therapy.

One question patients often ask is: "If I watch my PSA, how long will it be before the cancer spreads?" In fact, the cancer may have already spread but we can't find it! Recent studies suggest that the time from when a patient exhibits a biochemical failure following radical prostatectomy until they have documented metastatic disease is anywhere from five to eight years. There are many novel therapies such as Proscar and Eulexin or Proscar and Casodex which are available to treat this condition. Gene therapy is also being used.

Additionally, differentiation agents (which slow the growth of the cancer), antiangiogenesis (which affects blood vessels), and other compounds are being investigated for effectiveness in this setting. One strategy to consider is if the doubling time of these cancers can be extended by even small amounts, chances are the patient will die of something other than prostate cancer. In fact, stabilization of PSA by some of these novel methods is an important finding. It may not be necessary for the PSA to plummet to 0 for the patient to be considered "cured." In fact, stable disease is very important. There are thousands of men who are surviving with prostate cancer.

COST

Most of the men who are diagnosed with prostate cancer are older men. Medicare pays for a large number of the prostatectomies performed. The cost of health care has become very important. Insurance companies and HMOs are constantly looking for ways to reduce costs. A prostatectomy may cost $20,000 or more. Hospital costs can be a large portion of the total cost. A short time ago patients spent six or more days in the hospital. There have been several improvements in the surgical technique. Today many hospitals are sending the patients home within two or three days.

It is great when one can go home earlier. No one wants to be around a bunch of sick people. Besides, after a few days in the hospital, you would probably be sick of the food.☺

Chapter Nine
3D CONFORMAL RADIATION

*Drs. Gerald Hanks, Loren Buhle, Jeff Michalski,
Scott Press, and Aubrey Pilgrim*

X-rays are like a sharp knife that can reach inside the body and operate on a tumor without doing much damage to the surrounding tissues. It isusually much less traumatic and invasive than scalpel surgery. If this is so, why doesn't every one choose x-ray therapy? At one time persons treatedby x-ray therapy had more recurrences of cancer and also had a shorter life expectancy. X-ray technology and procedures have improved and most data now shows that there is very little, if any, differences in radical surgery and 3D conformal radiation therapy (3DCRT). Fig. 9-1 shows a 3D Conformal External Radiation machine.

Someone on the internet asked about skin damage during radiation. Dr. Loren Buhle, answered this way:

"When a linear accelerator is used to deliver radiation, the radiation beam has sufficient energy to begin depositing energy several centimeters below the skin surface. This distance between the skin surface and the depth where the x-ray beam starts depositing energy is called the "depth dose." This can be calculated during treatment planning.

Some men have erectile dysfunction or become impotent after the prostate is removed because the nerves and blood vessels that control erections are damaged or severed. These nerves and blood vessels may also be damaged by x-rays but may not be immediately evident. Certain tissues, such as the cells of blood vessels, which often divide and replace other cells, are more susceptible to x-rays than others.

The rate of impotence may be fairly low immediately following radiation. But over a period of time, the person may gradually lose his potency from the damage done to the blood vessels and nerves. He may also develop incontinence problems at some later date after radiation.

One disadvantage of x-rays is that it may not kill all of the cancer cells. Another disadvantage of radiation is that one can never be certain of the true pathological stage of the cancer. The clinical staging from biopsies, PSA and DRE is very often understaged. The only way to get a true pathological stage is after the prostate is removed.

HOW RADIATION KILLS CANCER CELLS

High dose radiation damages the DNA and chromosomes in the nucleus of cells. Unless the dose is very high, normal cells are usually able to recover. But cancer cells are less able to recover from radiation damage. They lose their ability to divide and multiply and eventually they die. All cells are more vulnerable to radiation during the process of dividing. Cancer cells usually divide more often than most normal cells so the radiation can kill more of them.

Cells that don't usually divide, such as the brain cells, are relatively immune to radiation. (Incidentally, we have several billion brain cells. Though not very sensitive to radiation, they are sensitive to certain chemicals such as alcohol. A few cells are killed every time we indulge. Other chemicals and drugs that we come in contact with also kills them off. As we get older, we become more absent-minded and forgetful as more of our brain cells are killed

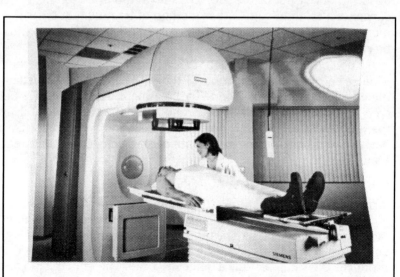

FIG. 9-1 A 3D Conformal External Radiation Machine

off. But we shouldn't worry about it too much. As a percentage of the total several billion, the few million or so that are killed off in a lifetime are a very small amount of our total. So go ahead and have a couple glasses of red wine. Enjoy. If you find yourself forgetting, just forget it.)

It is a paradox that a small dose of radiation to normal cells may cause them to become cancerous. It may not be enough to kill the cell, but it may damage some of the chromosomes and cause cancerous mutations. Dr. Malcolm Bagshaw, of Stanford, was one of the early pioneers in radiation. At one of his presentations he said that most healthy cells are able to repair any damage received during radiation but some of the damaged cells may eventually become cancerous. However, it may take several years for any such cancer to become significant. If the primary cancer is controlled, the patient may die of some other disorder before any x-ray-caused cancer would become a problem.

Some studies have indicated that neoadjuvant hormone therapy, that is, hormone therapy before radiation, may sensitize cancer cells so that radiation is more effective in killing them. Studies have also shown that adjuvant hormone therapy after radiation adds a survival advantage.

MAXIMUM DOSAGE

One disadvantage of radiation is that a person can only be exposed to about 6000 to 8000 rads maximum in a lifetime. If the cancer recurs, then some other method of treatment such as hormone therapy, salvage cryosurgery or a radical prostatectomy must be chosen.

If a person is to have 7000 rads (70 Gy) or more of x-ray therapy, it must be given over a period of time. The treatment is usually given five days a week. The usual treatment dose is two Gy per day. If a person is given 4 to 6 Gy at one time, it could be fatal, so the dose must be carefully controlled. If a person is given 2 Gy a day, their body can recover to some degree before the next treatment.

RADIATION TERMS AND ACRONYMS

Incidentally, there are some rather confusing terms and acronyms having to do with radiation. The term rad is an acronym meaning radiation absorbed dose. The term rem is an acronym for roentgen equivalent man. The rem is the absorbed dose of radiation that produces the same biological effect as 1 rad. The rem, the rad and the roentgen are all virtually the same. An example of a rem, for a routine chest x-ray, a person is exposed to about .1 to .2 rems. One hundred rads is equal to one gray (Gy). One gray is also equal to the same equivalent dose of ionizing radiation of 1 sievert (Sv). Another acronym is RBE which means relative biological effectiveness. The RBE is usually reserved for comparisons of heavy particle radiation. For instance, protons may have a RBE of 1, but neutrons may cause more damage and have a RBE of as much as 3. Normally, X-rays may have a RBE of less than 1.

A problem with earlier x-ray treatments for prostate cancer was that often the rectum and bladder were overexposed and severely damaged. Damage such as this usually required bladder and rectal surgery. After rectal or bladder surgery, the patient usually had to wear a colostomy bag to collect urine or feces. The procedures and technology have greatly improved and today there are very few cases where unwanted tissues are damaged during radiation.

One way they prevent damage to other tissues is by using shields and accurately directing the beams. They may also focus the beams over the left hip for a short time, then straight above the pelvic area, then from the right hip. The beams all intersect and focus on the prostate area, but since only a small amount of time is spent going through the hips and the bladder in front, little or no damage is done. Some systems use an x-ray machine that continuously moves from side to side to accomplish the same objective.

Most types of radiation are part of the electromagnetic spectrum that includes radio waves, infrared radiation, visible light, ultraviolet light, gamma rays and x-rays. There are two primary categories of radiation; ionizing and nonionizing. There are several different types of radiation for each of these categories. If you remember your high school science, all atoms have electrons in orbit around the nucleus. Ionizing means that the radiated beams are strong enough to forcibly dislodge electrons from their orbits. Once an atom loses an electron, it becomes ionized and now has an electric charge. Nonionizing radiation are things such as visible light, ultraviolet light, electromagnetic radio waves, microwaves, lasers and ultrasound. Nonionizing radiation may cause excitation of the atoms in molecules, but is not strong enough to dislodge electrons. Microwaves work by exciting and agitating the atoms in molecules which causes heat to be generated.

We are primarily interested in the ionizing type of radiation for prostate treatments, although there are several treatments that utilize lasers, microwaves and high frequency radio waves. There are three main types of ionizing radiation; x-rays, gamma rays and particle radiation. X-rays are generated artificially by special high voltage electrical machines. X-rays have no mass or weight or electrical charge. They have a very high frequency and a very short wavelength. Their penetrating power depends on the amount of energy or voltage used to create them. It requires about 100,000 volts to force x-ray beams to pass through a body for a normal x-ray image. For radiation therapy, it may require several million volts. With enough energy behind them, x-ray beams can even penetrate steel.

Gamma rays are very similar to x-rays except that they are produced by the spontaneous decay of radioactive materials such as uranium, plutonium, radium and certain radioactive isotopes. The radioactive materials activity is measured by their half-life. Plutonium has a half-life of 76 million years. At the end of 76 million years, exactly half of the plutonium's radioactivity would have been used up. Radium has a half-life of 1,622 years. There are several materials that can be made artificially radioactive due to bombardment with high energy particles. Palladium 103, used as seeds in brachytherapy, is an artificially produced radioactive isotope that has a half-life of 17 days.

There are several other artificially produced elements that have a half-life of only seconds or even microseconds. (Incidentally, as the radioactive materials decay, they lose weight and eventually become a different and lighter element. After several million years, uranium goes through several transformations into lesser atomic weight elements, including radium. After it loses all of its radioactivity, uranium becomes common lead.) There have been some tremendous advances in X-ray technology and treatments in the last few years.

The article below was written by Dr. Gerald Hanks, one of the country's foremost practitioners of 3DCRT.

THREE DIMENSIONAL CONFORMAL EXTERNAL BEAM TREATMENT OF PROSTATE CANCER

Gerald E. Hanks, M.D.

Chairman, Department of Radiation Oncology, Fox Chase Cancer Center

Introduction

Conformal three dimensional external beam treatment (3DCRT) of prostate cancer was introduced in the United States between 1987 and 1989 at the University of Michigan, Memorial Sloan Kettering Cancer Center and Fox Chase Cancer Center. Two of these three institutions then joined with 7 others (Univ. of California-San Francisco, Univ. of Chicago, Univ.

of Miami, Univ. of North Carolina, Univ. of Washington, Univ. of Wisconsin, and Washington University) in 1992 and began a prospective clinical trial group studying the effects of increased radiation dose in prostate cancer with 3DCRT. All of these institutions named above are considered as having substantial long term experience with 3DCRT.

The goal of 3DCRT is to "hit" all of the target (prostate) each day of treatment while hitting a minimum of surrounding normal tissue. Three steps are involved in assuring this level of accuracy:

(A) The patient is immobilized in an individual cast that assures that he is in the same position for his treatment planning and for each single treatment. The cast has been shown to reduce day-to-day variation in exactness of positioning for treatment by about 1 centimeter (cm). (Note: In case you don't remember your high school metric conversions, 1 cm is approximately 3/8 of an inch). The prostate, with or without seminal vesicles, can be included within a shell of normal tissue around the gland 1 cm thick. If immobilization is not used the shell of normal tissue around the gland would need to be 2 cm thick.

(B) A CT scan is performed with the patient in his cast and the prostate gland is identified in three dimensions.

(C) The treatment beams may be directed at the prostate from 4 to 6 directions. Each beam is specifically shaped so that it conforms to the shape of the target as seen from any particular beam direction. Conformal therapy is thus conforming the beam to the shape and size of the target while including a 1 cm margin of normal tissue for safety purposes.

The apex or bottom of the prostate gland is difficult to identify on a CT scan unless a urethrogram is performed. The urethrogram fills the penile urethra with dye up to the muscular urogenital diaphragm. The apex of the prostate has a fixed relationship to the urogenital diaphragm and that margin of the gland can be accurately included in conformal fields when this urethrogram technique is utilized.

What are the benefits of 3DCRT in reducing normal tissue injury?

Acute symptoms are those appearing during the course of radiation treatment and are markedly reduced by 3DCRT. Symptoms of bowel and bladder irritation that require medication were reduced from 57% to 36% of patients comparing 3DCRT patients to those treated with conventional treatment methods.

Late serious complications are dramatically reduced by 3DCRT and very few serious complications are observed even at doses that simply cannot be delivered with conventional treatment technology. Thus, patients can be treated to higher doses with an improved chance of curing their cancer while experiencing complications that are far below the USA national averages. When we compare the serious late complications of 3DCRT to previous reports of conventional radiation, 3DCRT has complications rates of less than 1% or 2% while conventional radiation may have a range from 5% to 10%.

Previous studies have demonstrated that patients with pretreatment PSAs higher than 10 ng/ml need radiation doses that are higher than commonly used to obtain optimal control of their cancers. A great deal of clinical research has been conducted by several of the institutions named above which indicates that 75 Gy improves the chances of controlling prostate cancer significantly more than the 65 Gy-70 Gy commonly used with conventional treatment.

What is the success of 3DCRT curing prostate cancer?

Our studies and those of the University of Michigan, Memorial Sloan Kettering Cancer Center and the University of California-San Francisco show 10 year results that are equal or better than those reported from prominent surgical series in patients with early disease (T1, T2A, B, Gleason 6 or less, PSA <10 ng/ml). Eighty-five percent of these patients will have no signs of cancer at 10 years. The results of 3DCRT in locally advanced cancers with higher PSAs stand alone as surgery is not generally performed in patients with bulky disease. Forty to 70% of these patients will have no signs of cancer at 10 years depending on pretreatment PSA characteristics.

At Fox Chase when we compared our 10-year results with 3DCRT to those previously obtained with conventional radiation therapy we noted an overall 10% improvement in biochemical freedom from cancer at 10 years.

Is surgery preferable for younger men?

We have recently examined our results in younger men because of the existing prejudice that surgery produces improved results in this group of patients. We found no such evidence as our men under 65 with pretreatment PSAs <10 ng/ml experience 80% biochemical freedom from disease at 10 years. This value is equal to treatment reports with surgery. In addition, we examined the maintenance of sexual potency in these young men. At 2.5-3 years after treatment 73% of them maintained their potency. This, again, is an excellent result that is superior to many surgical reports.

Thus, we feel that young men have a treatment option between conformal radiation therapy and radical prostatectomy and should be allowed to consider either of the two treatment options.

Our first 10-year results are available on favorable T2A patients with PSA <10 ng/ml, 80% are free of cancer at 10 years and are cured. Patients who survive 5 years without a rise in their PSA are also cured as we see only 2% of our total failures between 5 and 10 years.

ASTRO

The American Society for Therapeutic Radiology and Oncology (ASTRO) is the largest radiation oncology society in the world, with more than 5,000 members. As a leading organization in radiation oncology, biology and physics, the society's goals are to advance the scientific base of radiation therapy and to extend the benefits of radiation therapy to those with cancer.

Here is an abstract from a presentation made at the 1999 meeting of the American Society of Therapeutic Radiation Oncologists (ASTRO):

INTERMEDIATE OUTCOMES FOR 3D-CRT IN YOUNG MEN WITH NON-PALPABLE OR UNILOBAR PROSTATE CANCER AND PSA < 20 NG/ML

Mitro GC, Hanlon AL, Horwitz EM, Pinover WH, Hanks GE

Fox Chase Cancer Center, Philadelphia, PA, USA

Purpose:
   Young men with localized prostate cancer are more commonly treated with radical prostatectomy than radiotherapy. We report intermediate outcomes for young men treated with 3D conformal radiotherapy to see if this bias in treatment is supported by outcomes.

METHODS:
   Between 10/89 and 10/96, 96 men age 65 or younger with clinically staged T1-T2A (1997 AJCC), Gleason Score 2-6 without perineural invasion, pre-treatment PSA < 20 ng/ml adenocarcinoma of the prostate with a minimum follow-up of 2 years were treated at Fox Chase Cancer Center. All patients were treated with definitive 3D conformal external beam radiotherapy alone. The median follow-up was 46 months (24-

101 mos). The median patient age was 61years (51-65 yrs), and the median treatment dose was 7278 Gy (6780-7972 Gy).

Patients were stratified into groups depending on clinical stage (T1 vs. T2) and pre-treatment PSA (0-9.9 vs. 10-19.9 ng/ml). Estimates of rates for biochemical No Evidence of Disease (bNED) control and morbidity were calculated using the Kaplan-Meier product limit method. Biochemical failure was defined according to the ASTRO consensus definition and time was measured from the start of treatment. Genitourinary (GU) and gastrointestinal (GI) toxicity were assessed using the RTOG criteria.

Results:
Overall 5-year bNED control for all patients was 85%. The results appear durable, as no failure was noted after 40 months of follow-up. Grade 2 GU morbidity at 5 years was 5%, and no grade 3 GU morbidity was observed. Grade 2 GI morbidity at 5 years was 16%, and grade 3 GI morbidity at 5 years was 1%.

Conclusion:
Outcomes using 3D conformal external beam radiotherapy for the treatment of adenocarcinoma of the prostate in young patients who would be considered candidates for surgery or brachytherapy (clinical stage T1-T2, Gleason score 2-6, pre-treatment PSA 0-19.9 ng/ml) are excellent, suggesting that a treatment method bias based on age is not justified. Long-term morbidity is minimal, less than that documented in the majority of surgical series and equivalent to or better than those reported in most brachytherapy series.

Based on our results, young men have a choice of treatment for their early prostate cancer and should consider 3D-CRT.

SUMMARY

Three dimensional conformal radiation therapy is probably the most important technological advance in radiation oncology over the decade of the nineties. I believe that the reduction in serious side effects and the improvement in prostate cancer cure rates is of great importance. Men who are candidates for curative treatment now can consider the improved benefit associated with 3DCRT.

INTERNET QUESTIONS CONCERNING 3DCRT

Dr. Loren Buhle and Dr. Jeff Michalski are both experts on 3DCRT. They both spend a lot of time on the Internet answering questions.

Below are a couple of questions and answers:

Mr. P.S. wrote:

> "I am about to start high beam 3DCRT and have just yesterday completed the planning/simulation session wherein I was marked up, tatooed, x-rayed, and had a cat scan to verify the marking locations. My concern is that I have read in Dr. Michalski's home page that in most cases some sort of immobilization device is used to assure radiation pointing accuracy (I presume). In the trauma of the moment yesterday, I was too caught up to think to ask the following:
>
> How do the medical workers (doctor, dosemetrist, whoever) assure that the radiation is going to be positioned in the place that they would like?"

Answer by Dr. Loren Buhle:

> There are laser alignment aids in the room (look along the walls, you'll see them). This gets the patient's body in the right place. Then there may be immobilization casts to get the body in the right position. Of course, if you tense your buttocks, the bladder/prostate move...though your body is in the same position.During the delivery of the radiation...a film is sometimes taken (this is called a portal image). In one or two places, a camera is used instead of film and a movie is taken during treatment (this is a research setting only). The purpose of this portal view is to compare with the simulation films. Remember...the target consists of a boundary of normal tissue at risk...so if there is a bit of motion, say a few millimeters, it won't matter anyway.
>
> The CT scan was to collect contiguous image sections to generate a three dimensional model of your body (organs, tumor and surrounding normal tissue at risk). Depending on the treatment planning session...this model is used to visualize the radiation portals and (might be) used to calculate the radiation treatment (dose deposition). I wrote code while at Penn to take into account the heterogeneity of the tissue in the beam path...since the energy deposition differs when the beam goes through airspace, liquid, bone, and soft tissue. Is this important in the outcome? I'd like to say yes...but I really don't know (probably more important where there is a lot of heterogeneity...such as treating lung tumors).
>
> Very likely they will use the tattoos for lining your body up with the lasers in the room...and the rest of the positioning will be confirmed with films taken during the treatments.
>
> "Generally, how many workers (one?) are involved in the actual treatment process on a day-to-day basis, for a forty-treatment series extending over eight weeks?"
>
> There is the physician, the planning personnel (dosimetrist, medicalphysicist), technicians delivering the treatment, and the nurses.

Here is Dr. Jeff Michalski's answer:

In 3DCRT the CAT scan is the critical first element for tumor localization and plan development. It would not be used to "verify" markings. Markings should be determined "FROM" the CAT data. In 3D planning methods the CAT scan serves as the initial planning simulation session. We may use a "verification simulation" after the planning to verify markings. This is done in a conventional therapy simulator.

Dr. Loren answered your question about positioning but I think it is worth restating that modern day linacs are checked for accuracy to within 2mm and a series of laser alignment devices in the room assist in the patient set up. Therapy portal radiographs (port films or port images) are compared to the original prescription image (simulation film or digital reconstructed radiograph from the 3D planning system) to assure accurate setup. Standard procedure is to check these weekly.

On our 3D dose escalation trial we check them twice weekly for the first week or two. In addition, in creating the RT plan, the physician should have allowed for some variation in the position of the target. The margin for uncertainty accounts for small setup errors and internal organ motion.

The immobilization device we use is a foam cradle ("alpha cradle" tm). Some investigators have shown the use of a device like this minimizes the variability of treatment setup. Other institutions use thermally sensitive plastic devices. These soften when warmed and firm up as they cool. They are heated and then molded to the patients' contour.

As to the number of workers in the room, there are always at least two radiotherapists (RTT) involved in the setup procedure. On many of our 3DCRT patients, we use 3 RTT's. During the course of 8 weeks we try to keep the same team together, but invariably there will be some "cross coverage" or team rotation to keep each RTT familiar with the setup and procedure for the 3DCRT patients.

JEFF M. MICHALSKI, M.D. Radiation Oncology Center, Mallinckrodt Institute of Radiology, Washington University, St. Louis, MO.

NOCTURIA

Here is a question on the Internet about a 3DCRT complication:

Three months into CHB and 3 weeks into 3DCRT. Most difficult side effect is nocturia. About every 2 hours after going to bed. During day I am totally normal. Tried several prescriptions, nothing helps. Now for the wild idea. What if I took a diuretic during the day to produce an empty bladder by bedtime? If my bladder is empty would that reduce the need to urinate every 2 hours during sleep time? Appreciate any comments by anybody. H.G.

Answer by Dr. Scott Press:

The nocturia that you are feeling is related to the radiation therapy, not the presence of large amounts of urine in your bladder. Since RT causes inflammation in the trigone (base) portion of the bladder and the prostatic urethra as a natural side effect, the nerves there are very sensitive. The slightest amount of urine will cause you to feel that you have to urinate i.e. 50 cc. At night a buildup of a small amount of urine makes it feel like you have to go. The treatments for this condition, known as "urgency," are not totally effective.

I can tell you one that will not work and that is to take a diuretic during the day. This will only increase the symptoms by causing large amounts of urine to be produced at a time. Therapy revolves around the etiology of the symptoms.

If the urgency is caused primarily by the prostate, try Hytrin 5 mg every night or Cardura 4 mg every night. These drugs are known as alpha-1 blockers and inhibit the nerves causing symptoms in the prostate. If the urgency is primarily bladder in origin: Ditropan 5 mg at night time will calm the bladder muscle and nerves down so that the feeling of urgency will be less.

Anti-inflammatory meds like Naprosyn, Aleve, or Advil will help also but carry a risk of bleeding since they inhibit platelet aggregation.

Hope this helps.

Scott M. Press, M.D. Department of Urology, The Long Island Jewish Medical Center, New Hyde Park, New York 11040

RADIATION PLUS HORMONE SUPPRESSION

Dr. Gerald Hanks has also done some studies combining hormone suppression therapy with radiation. He reported the results of a study at the American Society of Clinical Oncologists (ASCO) 2000 meeting. Here is a copy of his abstract #1284:

RTOG Protocol 92-02: A Phase III Trial of the Use of Long Term Androgen Suppression Following Neoadjuvant Hormonal Cytoreduction and Radiotherapy in Locally Advanced Carcinoma of the Prostate. Gerald E. Hanks, Jiandong Lu, Mitchell Machtay, Varagur Venkatesan, Wayne Pinover, Roger Byhardt, Seth A Rosenthal, Fox Chase Cancer Ctr, Philadelphia, PA; American Coll of Radiology, Philadelphia, PA; Univ of Pennsylvania, Philadelphia, PA; Univ of Western Ontario, London, Canada; Medical Coll of Wisconsin, Milwaukee, WI; Sutter Cancer Ctr, Sacramento, CA.

RTOG Protocol 92-02 was a prospective randomized trial of androgen suppression and external beam radiation in patients with locally advanced prostate cancer (T2C-T4) with PSAs less than 150 ng/ml. All patients received Zoladex and Flutamide two months before and two months during radiation and were randomized to no further therapy or 24 months of additional Zoladex alone. Of 1554 patients entered, 34 were found to be ineligible. The median follow-up is 4.8 years. The two arms were well matched on stratification and other variables.

The group with long-term androgen deprivation (LTAD) showed significant improvement in disease-free survival 54% vs 34% (p = .0001), local progression 6% vs 13% (p = .0001), distant metastasis 11% vs 17% (p = .001) and biochemical failure 21% vs 46% (p = .0001). Fifty-four patients died of prostate cancer in the short-term androgen deprivation group (STAD) compared to 33 in the LTAD. Disease specific survival (DSS) showed a trend in favor of the LTAD group 92% vs 87% (p = .07). Five-year survival was not different between the two arms (78% vs 79%). There was a significant increase in RTOG grade 3 and 4 bowel complications in the LTAD group, 42 vs 26 (p = .04).

Two other subsets were analyzed; one comparable to those entered in Bolla et al, NEJM 1998. This subset (T3, T4 and T2 with Gleason 8-10) showed no survival difference (77% vs 79%) at 5 years but a significant advantage in DSS for LTAD 90% vs 86% (p = .03). The second subset, including all Gleason 8-10, is compared to a previous subset analysis of RTOG 85-31 (Pilepich, JCO, 1997).

Five-year survival was significantly better with LTAD 80% vs 69% (p = .02). DSS was significantly better with LTAD 90% vs 78% (p = .007). In Gleason 8-10 tumors, 29 patients died of prostate cancer in the STAD vs 12 in the LTAD. A survival advantage is observed for LTAD in the subset of Gleason 8-10 T2C to T4 tumors with PSA < 150 ng/ml, and a DSS advantage is observed for the subset including all T3,4 or T2 Gleason 8-10 tumors.

This study supports the continued use and study of LTAD in patients with poorly differentiated or locally advanced prostate cancers.

Another study was conducted by the European Organization for Research and Treatment of Cancer (EORTC) Radiotherapy Cooperative Group. Results of the study showed that with a median follow-up of 61 months, overall survival rates for Zoladex with radiotherapy were significantly increased from 62 percent to 78 percent, and disease-free survival rates were increased from 40 percent to 75 percent, when compared to the radiotherapy alone group.[1]

For some time there has been an upper limit of about 70 Gray that can be administered. But new techniques and instruments can now safely deliver doses up to 78 Gy or more. A study of 149 patients who received a radiation dose of 70 Gy was compared to 151 patients who received 78 Gy. Forty-eight percent of the patients who received 70 Gy did not have rising PSA levels five years after treatment but 75 percent of those who received 78 Gy did not have a rising PSA.

INTENSITY MODULATED RADIATION THERAPY

Intensity modulated radiation therapy (IMRT) is a safe way to accurately deliver high doses of radiation to the prostate while preserving normal tissue nearby, a new study shows. A study of 171 patients with early stage prostate cancer compared three-dimensional conformal radiation therapy (3D CRT) to intensity modulated radiation therapy (IMRT). The study found that when the radiation oncologists used either of the two techniques, higher doses of radiation (81 Gy) could be used without significant urinary side effects. However, IMRT was more effective in avoiding the rectum and surrounding area. The risk of rectal bleeding two years after treatment was two percent for IMRT compared to 10 percent for conventional 3D CRT.

The IMRT system is produced by the Nomos Company at http://www.nomos.com.

There are several centers now using IMRT. One of the centers is the Cancer Treatment Centers of America—Call 1-800-788-8485 ext. 5170 for more information.

RISING PSA

Radiation therapy is commonly employed to treat localized prostate cancer. Since the prostate remains and can be a source of PSA, there exists a great deal of debate in describing what constitutes failure. Several recent publications suggest that following successful external beam radiation or seed implants, patients who remain free of disease have an almost undetectable PSA level. There seems to be little argument that once the PSA begins to rise from a baseline level (called nadir level), that this constitutes failure. There are many things to consider when faced with a patient who exhibits a rising PSA after failed local therapy.

There is some evidence that there may be a PSA "bounce" within two years or so after radiation, with either external or seed implants. The PSA may go to a very low level and stay there for some time, but then it may rise unexpectedly for a short time. This rise can be frightening, but in many cases it falls back down to a low nadir in a short time. However, if the PSA continues to rise, then it should be a matter of concern.

Since the person still has prostatic tissue, it will produce a certain amount of PSA. There is some evidence that some of the tissue may recover from the radiation and begin growing again. Because of this the ultrasensitive PSA tests are of little benefit.

A ProstaScint test may be able to detect any metastatic colonies. If so, then additional radiation may able to destroy the colony. This treatment could only be used if the man has not had the radiation limit.

Usually hormone therapy would be the treatment of choice after radiation failure. If this does not control the PSA, it may be necessary to use chemotherapy.

Chapter Ten
PROTON BEAM RADIATION

By Drs. Carl Rossi, Jr. and Aubrey Pilgrim

Particle radiation has weight and mass and usually an electrical charge. X-rays and gamma rays have no weight or mass. Particle radiation includes parts of atoms such as positively charged protons and neutral neutrons. Massive cyclotrons and linear accelerators use enormous amounts of energy to accelerate these particles. Protons and neutrons have a mass that is 1800 times that of electrons so they cannot be accelerated to the same speed as electrons or beta particles. Since most particles have a charge, they can be aimed and controlled by electronic means. Neutrons do not have a charge so they cannot be controlled as accurately as the charged particles, but they are used because they actually have a higher relative biological effectiveness (RBE) than other particles.

Since x-rays and gamma rays have no weight or mass, they can travel very fast, approaching the speed of visible light, or 186,000 miles per second. Scientists would like to be able to get the same speed from particles, but since they are quite heavy and massive, it is not possible.

UNDERSTANDING HOW PROTONS WORK

All matter is made up of atoms. This includes animal, vegetable, mineral and metals. It also includes cancerous tumors. In the center of every atom is a nucleus. Orbiting the nucleus of each atom are negatively charged electrons.

When energized charged particles, such as protons or other forms of radiation, pass near orbiting electrons, the positive charge of the protons attracts the negatively charged electrons, pulling them out of their orbits. This is called ionization; it changes the characteristics of the atom and consequently the character of the molecule within which the atom resides.

This crucial change is the basis for the beneficial aspects of all forms of radiation therapy. Because of ionization, the radiation damages molecules within the cells, particularly the DNA or genetic material. Damaging the DNA destroys specific cell functions, especially the ability to divide or proliferate.

Enzymes within the cells attempt to rebuild the injured area of the DNA; however, if damage from the radiation is too extensive, the enzymes will not be able to repair the injury.

While both normal and cancerous cells go through this repair process, a cancer cell's ability to repair molecular injury is frequently inferior. As a result, cancer cells sustain more permanent damage and subsequent cell death than occurs in the normal cell population. This permits selective destruction of bad cells that may be growing among good cells.

Both conventional x-ray therapy and proton beams work on the principle of selective cell destruction. The major advantage of proton treatment over conventional radiation, however, is that the characteristic energy distribution of protons can be deposited in tissue volumes designated by the physician in a three-dimensional pattern. This capability provides greater control and precision and, therefore, superior management of treatment.

Radiation therapy requires that conventional x-rays be delivered into the body in total doses sufficient to assure that enough ionization events occur to damage all the cancer cells. The lack of charge and mass in conventional x-rays, which are called photons, results in most of the energy being deposited in normal tissues near the body's surface. Undesirable energy may be deposited beyond the target or the cancer volume as the x-rays continue through the tissue.

This undesirable pattern of energy placement can result in unnecessary damage to healthy tissues. This may prevent the use of sufficient radiation to control the cancer. There is a finite limit as to how much radiation the body can withstand.

PROTONS ENERGIZED TO SPECIFIC VELOCITIES

Protons may be energized to specific velocities. These energies determine how deeply in the body protons will deposit their maximum energy. As the protons move through the body, they slow down, causing increased interaction with orbiting electrons.

Maximum interaction with electrons occurs as the protons approach their targeted stopping point. Thus, maximum energy is released within the designated cancer volume. The surrounding healthy cells receive significantly less injury than the cells in the designated volume. This point, where the high dosage region of energy release occurs, is called the Bragg peak.

The favorable absorption characteristics of protons allows the physician to predict and control their depth of travel within the patient. At the tumor site, the Bragg peak can be enlarged to conform to the thickness of the designated volume of the tumor. The heavy mass also results in minimal deviation and minimal side-scatter. This is a significant factor in reducing unwanted side-effects and maximizing treatment benefit.

CONVENTIONAL X-RAYS

Conventional x-rays lose most of their energy near the body's surface and exponentially deposit energy as they travel through tissue. Electrons, because of their low mass, are easily deflected from their initial direction and produce significant secondary lateral scatter. When photons or electrons (x-rays) are used, healthy tissues surrounding the tumor target frequently receive equal doses, given the designated volume. Radiation oncologists attempt to circumvent these problems. They often employ multi-field arrangements to build up the doses and spare as much of the normal tissue as possible, by restricting the dose in those tissues to a level the patient can tolerate.

Multi-field arrangements can be used with protons also. When they are used, the dose to normal tissues is cut to half or less, thereby minimizing adverse, normal-tissue damage. When multiple proton fields are used, the dose in the overlapped beams is further increased relative to normal tissue. This permits more effective doses to be delivered to the designated volume than can be achieved with x-rays.

Because of the dose-distribution characteristic of protons, the radiation oncologist can increase the dose to the tumor while reducing the dose to surrounding normal tissues. This allows the dose to be increased beyond that which less-conformal radiation would allow. The overall affects lead to the potential for fewer harmful side effects, more direct impact on the tumor, and increased tumor control.

The patient feels nothing during treatment. The minimized normal-tissue injury results in the potential for fewer effects following treatment such as nausea, vomiting, or diarrhea. The patient experiences a better quality of life during and after proton treatment. Protons provide a vast new potential for non-invasive treatment of all cancer patients when the tumor is localized.

For conformal proton beam planning purposes the patients are immobilized in a custom-fitting plastic cylinder. A balloon is placed in the rectum and inflated with 120 cc of water so as to exclude the majority of the rectal volume from the prostate treatment fields. A thin slice Computed Tomography (CT) scan of the pelvis is performed with the patient in his immobilization cylinder. The prostate, bladder, and rectum are outlined by a physician on LLUMC's 3D conformal planning system which utilizes beam's eye view planning and dose-volume histograms to optimize individual treatment plans.

In virtually all instances a simple two field (right and left lateral beams) plan provides for the best coverage of the gland while sparing the majority of the bladder and rectum. All individual cerrobend apertures and wax tissue compensators are produced on automated milling machines controlled by the 3D planning system. Patient position is verified daily before each conformal proton beam treatment by obtaining orthogonal radiographs of the patient's pelvis in the treatment position via a coaxially mounted x-ray tube. Measurements are made from various bony landmarks to the isocenter and compared with optimal measurements obtained from a computer-generated digitally reconstructed radiograph (generated from the CT planning scan). The treatment table is moved to match the various measurements.

Typically, the time required for each patient's set-up and treatment is 20-30 minutes per day.

Between January 1992 and December 1995, 260 patients with early stage prostate cancer (defined as stages T1-T2B, PSA <15 NO or Nx, no prior hormonal therapy or surgery) were treated. The radiation dose to the prostate was 74-75CGE (Cobalt Gray Equivalent, utilizing a proton RBE of 1.1) given at a dose rate of 1.8-2.0 Gy per day. Two hundred and nine patients were treated with conformal protons alone while fifty one were treated with a combination of 30 CGE protons to the prostate and seminal vesicles plus 45 GY conformal photons to the pelvis.

By 1998 the number of patients treated had risen to 319. Their study was published in Urology 53: 978-984 1999.

Three hundred nineteen patients with T1—T2b prostate cancer and initial prostate-specific antigen (PSA) levels of 15.0 ng/mL or less received conformal radiation doses of 74 to 75 cobalt gray equivalent with protons alone or combined with photons. No patient had pre- or post-treatment hormonal therapy until disease progression was documented. Patients were evaluated for biochemical disease-free survival, PSA nadir, and toxicity; the mean and median follow-up period was 43 months.

Overall 5-year clinical and biochemical disease-free survival rates were 97% and 88%, respectively. Initial PSA level, stage, and post-treatment PSA nadir were independent prognostic variables for biochemical disease-free survival: a PSA nadir 0.5 ng/mL or less was associated with a 5-year biochemical disease-free survival rate of 98%, versus 88% and 42% for nadirs 0.51 to 1.0 and greater than 1.0 ng/mL, respectively. No severe treatment-related morbidity was seen.

It appears that patients treated with conformal protons have 5-year biochemical disease-free survival rates comparable to those who undergo radical prostatectomy, and display no significant toxicity.

Protons are a superior particle for clinical use because:

They have favorable physical dose absorption characteristics in tissues which allow exact energy deposition, thereby sparing normal tissues and organs,

Their radiobiologic characteristics are similar to photons (x-rays), and thus, are well known.

As of November 1999, 4,666 patients have been treated at Loma Linda for several different types of cancer. Proton Beam therapy seems to have similar results as that attained from Conformal 3D radiation.

As of April 2001, over 1200 prostate cancer patients have been treated at Loma Linda. They now have 7 years of data. When compared, stage by stage, with surgery, it appears that proton beam therapy is equivalent to surgery.

If you are considering proton treatment at Loma Linda, you or your physician should contact the patient referral office:

Phone: (909) 558-4288 or (800) PROTONS (USA only)

Fax: (909) 558-4829

E-mail: Referral@dominion.llumc.edu—referral and information service

For more information, visit their web site at: http://www.llu.edu/llu/ci/

Chapter Eleven
BRACHYTHERAPY
Seed Therapy For Localized Prostate Cancer And High Dose Rate Brachytherapy

By Drs. Haakon Ragde, Gordon Grado, Frank Critz, Hamilton Williams and Stephen Doggett for seeds and Nisar Syed, Ajmel Puthawala and Aubrey Pilgrim for HDR

This chapter covers the seed implantation (SI) of radioactive pellets or seeds into the prostate. The temporary or High Dose Rate (HDR) procedure will also be covered. These procedures are very popular and there are several sites that perform SI and HDR. Some of the sites use procedures that are slightly different than others. However, they all seem to have similar success rates.

INTRODUCTION
Conceptually, the goal of treating a cancerous tumor anywhere in the body should be twofold: to cure the cancer and minimize negative impacts on quality of life. In the U.S. the mainstays of treatment for prostate cancer confined to the gland itself have been surgical removal and traditional external beam radiation. We believe that brachytherapy or seed implants is a good alternative to surgery or external beam radiation in selected patients.

WHAT IS PROSTATE BRACHYTHERAPY?
Prostate brachytherapy (also called seed therapy, seed implantation, or interstitial radiation) treats prostate cancer by placing radioactive seeds via needles directly into the gland. This allows the delivery of a highly confined dose of radiation directly to the prostate, sparing adjacent healthy tissue from radiation injury, and reducing side effects and complications.

"*Brachy-*" comes from the Greek word meaning "short" and is used to describe treatment with radioactive sources or materials placed at a short distance to the tumor in comparison to "*tele-*"

(therapy) which refers to external radiation treatments delivered at a distance from the patient and the tumor.

In the late 1980s sophisticated computerized imaging and dosimetry techniques were developed. These techniques permitted correct radiation dose calculation and precise seed placements. Fig. 11-1 is a drawing of an ultrasound-guided seed implant. The ultrasound probe is inserted in the rectum which provides visualization of the prostate and the seed placement.

In the mid 1980s, Palladium–103 (Pd^{103}), a radioisotope that promised a more aggressive attack on the cancer, became available for needle insertion. The first implantation with this radioisotope was performed by Dr. Ragde in 1987.

Most of the preliminary work-up is performed in a physician's office, and only the actual implant requires a surgical facility. In most centers today the procedure is performed on a cost-effective outpatient or overnight hospital stay, and most patients are able to resume their normal daily activities within 24 to 48 hours.

With a general consensus that PSA measurements after any form of prostate cancer treatment are the most effective way to detect persistence or recurrence of the cancer, no specific treatment

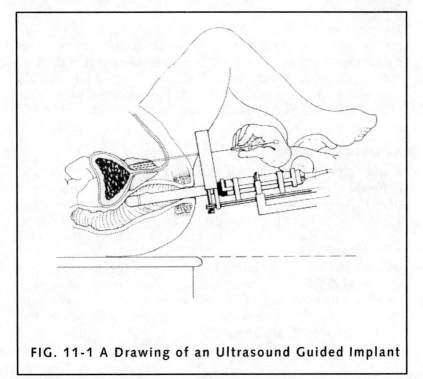

FIG. 11-1 A Drawing of an Ultrasound Guided Implant

method today can lay claim to long-term (15 year) results; the PSA assay has been in clinical usefor fewer than ten years. In other words, results with prostate brachytherapy, surgery, and external radiation all are limited to fewer than ten years of PSA follow-up. Ten-year data, using serum PSA determinations and repeat needle biopsies as determinants show prostate brachytherapy cure rates equal to the best surgical cure rates reported, but with fewer complications.

WHO ARE APPROPRIATE CANDIDATES FOR SEED THERAPY?

Seed therapy alone will only provide effective radiation to the prostate and a five millimeter-wide surrounding margin. In some patients, who have larger and more aggressive cancers, there is a risk of tumor spread beyond the prostate into the surrounding area. As a result, these patients are not good candidates for interstitial radiation alone. A combination treatment consisting of radioactive seeds and external beam radiation may better address the issue of this "possible locally advanced" disease.

WHAT DOES PROSTATE SEED THERAPY INVOLVE?

Consultation:

Seed therapy is a team effort, involving both a urologist and a radiation oncologist. They will review the patient's records, discuss the different treatments available, consider the complications and costs (quality-of-life costs as well as dollars-and-cents) associated with each treatment, so that the patient and his family can make the best decision based on age, health and life style preference.

Patient Evaluation:

A careful physical exam and review of the patient's records are performed to get a reasonable assurance that the cancer is confined to the prostate. Several additional tests may be required, such as CT scan (to look for evidence of cancer outside the prostate), Urinary Flow Study (a test that measures how well the bladder empties) and Cystoscopy (use of an instrument to look inside the bladder and urethra to further evaluate bladder emptying.)

A more detailed diagnostic ultrasound of the prostate may be required to evaluate the position of the prostate tumor in the gland, as well as to note any surgical cavity left from previous prostate surgery (such as a TURP).

Additional tests are usually required, such as routine preoperative bloodwork, chest x-ray, and an electrocardiogram. These will aid the anesthesiologist in determining the patient's ability to receive anesthesia.

Personalized Treatment Plan:

This step consists of making a geometric map of the prostate that is derived from an ultrasound scan. This map, also known as a "volume study," forms the basis for an individual patient's treatment plan and is key to a successful implant. It shows the exact volume and shape of the gland, as well as the proposed seed locations. The map is entered into a planning computer to construct a three-dimensional implant model. It also prescribes individual seed strengths, and specifies precise intra-prostatic seed positions, to make certain that the whole gland will be effectively radiated and that the adjacent healthy tissue is spared from radiation injury.

Depending on the width of the bony pubic arch or equipment limitation, prostate glands may need to be reduced before treatment. This may take two to three months, and is readily accomplished by medication that temporarily shuts off testosterone production, to inhibit the cancerous growth and simultaneously shrink the size of the gland. Without pubic arch obstruction we have implanted prostate volumes up to 210 cubic centimeters.

What Radioactive Sources (Seeds) Are Used?

Most commonly Palladium-103 and Iodine-125 (I^{125}) are used. Both are contained in tiny titanium casings which the body can tolerate long-term. Both types of radioactive seeds give off low energy X-rays, with most of the radioactivity released within a short period of time: Palladium 103 in 3 months, and Iodine 125 in 6 months. The main difference between them is the half-life and rate of radiation delivery. Although there is no clinical evidence that one is more effective than the other, some physicians prefer to use Palladium for more aggressive cancers, or select the radioactive isotope based on gland size or shape, or on the basis of past therapy or surgery.

After the seeds are inserted into the prostate they will remain there permanently. Since only a small volume of prostate tissue is radiated by each seed, many seeds have to be inserted to cover the entire gland. This is important because microscopic cancer cells may be present at different sites within the gland even though the biopsy in the general area may have been negative. The number of seeds implanted into the prostate for treatment may vary from 40 to well over 100, depending on the size of the gland.

Although the cumulative effect of the seeds results in high-dose radiation to the gland, the low energy and short tissue penetration of the radioisotopes protect adjacent normal organs and tissue from radiation injury.

Performing the Implant:

The actual implant is usually performed in a surgical facility and takes about an hour to complete. It is most commonly done under spinal anesthesia although general anesthesia may also be used, depending on the preference of the anesthesiologist and the patient.

An ultrasound probe with an attached template guiding device corresponding to the grid on the ultrasound screen, is inserted into the rectum. Video-imaging from the ultrasound is used to guide the insertion of each needle through the perineum into its computer-designated position in the prostate. Each hollow needle may contain several seeds. The individual seeds are then ejected along the path of the needle as it is slowly withdrawn.

When the implant procedure is completed, proper placement is verified by taking an x-ray of the lower abdomen. Before leaving the operating room, a catheter is placed in the patient's bladder to drain the urine.

The Recovery Room:

After the implant the patient will go to the Recovery Room, where he will remain until the effects of anesthesia have worn off. The catheter is usually removed within 24 hours, but it may sometimes be necessary to leave it in longer.

Follow-up Instructions:

Postoperative instructions, covering medications and appointments are given before the patient leaves the treatment facility. Generally there is very little discomfort after the implant, but pain medication is available should it be needed.

Radiation Precaution:

Palladium and Iodine are low energy radioactive isotopes. This means that most of the radiation is shielded by the prostate itself. What little escapes beyond the gland is insignificant and not considered a risk for most people. Small children and pregnant women, however, may be more sensitive to the effects of radiation, and intimate contact, such as hugging and sitting on the patient's lap, should be avoided for the first two months following an Iodine implant and for one month following a Palladium implant.

Short-term Side-effects:

Side effects, consisting of some urinary frequency and urgency, and possibly some burning on voiding, are not unusual after the implant. They are caused by the radiation from the seeds in the prostate, and the symptoms may last from a few days to several weeks.

Long-term Side-effects:

Incontinence and impotence, the most dreaded complications associated with treatments intended to cure prostate cancer, occur less frequently after brachytherapy than following surgical removal of the prostate or traditional radiation treatment. The observed impotency rate after seed therapy depends on the patient's age: For those patients who were potent before treatment, and did not receive external beam radiation, those less than 60 years were still potent after treatment; for ages between 60 and 70 years, 20% had erectile dysfunction (ED); above 70 years old between 35 to 50% had ED.

There should be no incontinence if the patient has not had previous surgery of his prostate such as transurethral resection of the prostate (TURP).

CLINICAL RESULTS

As mentioned, PSA is a key indicator in monitoring response to treatment for prostate cancer. Elevation of PSA after treatment may indicate failure to eradicate the cancer, although it may also indicate the presence of metastatic disease. PSA levels may denote the presence of cancer several years before it can be detected on clinical exams. When the prostate is removed surgically, PSA in the serum rapidly decreases to undetectable levels. The radiated prostate, however, continues to produce PSA, but at very low levels.

Dr. Ragde's group in Seattle has reported on 229 consecutive (unselected) brachytherapy patients followed for 12 years. During that time period only 4 patients died from prostate cancer, yielding a cancer-specific survival rate of 98%. This compares favorably with prostate cancer-specific survival rates reported from surgical centers, which range from 83-98%.

In marked contrast to the treatment and recovery times required for surgery and external beam radiation, seed implantation is performed as a one-day outpatient procedure, or—in some cases—as an overnight hospital stay. Most patients are back to their usual daily activities in a day or two.

With a total price tag of about half the cost of a radical prostate-ctomy, seed therapy should provide substantial saving for patients and third party payers alike.

HAAKON RAGDE, M.D. and GORDON L. GRADO, M.D. have merged their practices. They have offices in Seattle, Washington at:

10330 Meridian Ave. N. Suite 300, Seattle, WA 98133

206-729-2266Fax 206-729-0309

In Scottsdale, Arizona

2926 N. Civic Center Plaza, Scottsdale, AZ 85251, 480-614-6300

And also in Des Moines, Iowa.

Call (800) 622-7814 for more information about any of the offices.

DR. STEPHEN DOGGETT'S PROTOCOL

Dr. Stephen Doggett practices in the Los Angeles area. He invited me, Aubrey, to observe the seeding of one of his patients.

Before the seeding process a plan had been formulated. This plan was based on the clinical diagnosis and ultrasound images. Just before the seeding, he uses a sophisticated software program called an image registered intra-operative real time treatment plan-ning (IRIRTP) for permanent seed prostate brachytherapy.

Under computer control, the ultrasound provides 5mm image slices of the prostate. The Interplantâ IRIRTP from Burdette Medical Systems, Inc. allows the ultrasound images to be entered into the treatment planning computer. Optical probe registration permits precise localization of the ultrasound probe to the template and prostate. Prostate size is precisely documented and errors intro-duced by prostatic motion are mitigated. The treatment plan is then automatically generated in the operating room on a PC.

Automatic optimization minimizes operator input. Interplant IRIRTP allows real time, pre-implant, three-dimensional superim-position of translucent isodose surfaces over the prostatic anatomy for a simulated micro-dosimetric analysis of radiation exposure to any point in the prostate and surrounding structures.

During the pre-planning stage, Dr. Doggett had determined that he would use 84 PD[103] seeds. The seeds were placed on the images in the computer. The computer then calculated the placement and dosage of each seed. This prevented any cold spots that were not getting enough radiation. It also calculated the amount of dosage that the urethra and rectal tissue would receive. These computer calculations allowed for the optimum placement of the seeds. Some brachytherapists use long hollow needles that have been pre-loaded with up to 10 or more seeds. These needles are inserted into the prostate, and using the ultrasound image, the seeds are then pushed out at specific areas as the needle is withdrawn.

Another system is to place hollow needles in the prostate at areas according to the plan.

The cartridges mount on a Mick applicator. The Mick applicator is attached to one of the hollow needles. A long thin wire is used to push a seed into place in the prostate. As the wire is withdrawn, another seed drops down and it is pushed into place. Each seed is placed according to the planned image on the computer screen. The entire procedure took about 45 minutes. The patient had been given a tranquilizer and slept through the entire process.

Burdette Medical Systems says that the Interplant IRIRTP is the first significant technological advance in prostate permanent seed brachytherapy in 15 years. Interplantâ IRIRTP is designed to substantially reduce human operator input during the treatment planning process with its attendant error rate. Inaccuracies due to prostatic motion and size changes in the time between planning and surgery are mitigated.

Dr. Stephen Doggett has an office at 14642 Newport Ave #470 Tustin, CA 92780 . Tel. 714-669-4019.

RADIOTHERAPY CLINICS OF GEORGIA (RCOG)

By Drs. Frank Critz and Hamilton Williams

The physicians of the Radiotherapy Clinics of Georgia in Atlanta (http://www.prostRcision.com) have specialized in the treatment of prostate cancer since 1977, beginning the retropubic (open) implantation. When it became apparent in 1979 that the old style retropubic technique was ineffective in curing prostate cancer, Dr, Frank Critz, founder of the clinic, began development of simultaneous irradiation, that is, prostate implant followed by conformal external irradiation. During the next 5 years the technique was refined, and in 1984 RCOG began a formal study of simultaneous irradiation which continues to this day.

In 1992, RCOG changed from the retropubic technique to the transperineal ultrasound guided technique. With the improved seed distribution allowed by the transperineal technique we were able to double the dose of radiation given to the prostate with a greater margin of safety than could be achieved with the open technique. We now have treated more than 3,000 men with prostate cancer with simultaneous irradiation, amassing the greatest amount of experience and results in the United States in the process.

While the approach of simultaneous irradiation, performing the implant first then using the seeds as a target for conformal external beam irradiation, made logical sense, it was when PSA was made available for clinical use in 1987 that its true value became apparent. Even in the 1990s, most physicians believed that as long as the PSA was within the normal range after radiotherapy, the patient was cancer free. However, Dr. Critz noted early on that men treated with simultaneous irradiation achieved PSAs not just in the normal range, but they achieved undetectable levels, the same as disease-free men achieve after surgery. Even more importantly, the overwhelming majority of men who achieved these undetectable levels remained cancer-free.

RCOG has pursued a consistent approach for men with prostate cancer since 1984: implant followed by simultaneous conformal irradiation, a process called *prostRcision*. ProstRcision means "excision of the prostate by radiation," and is called such because the men treated with this technique achieve and maintain undetectable PSA levels, 0.2 ng/ml or less, just as often as men treated with radical prostatectomy. In effect, prostRcision is a "radiation prostatectomy," but without the damage to the urination muscles and the sex nerves that happens so often with surgery.

Using the identical nadir goal as required after surgery, achievement and maintenance of PSA nadir £ 0.2 ng/ml, the 10 and 15 year results of prostRcision are identical to those of Dr. Walsh's radical prostatectomy series.

In conclusion, Radiotherapy Clinics of Georgia offers a unique, time proven approach to prostate cancer backed up by a program of rigorous, ongoing research. We encourage any man with prostate cancer to investigate RCOG.

You can contact the RCOG at (404) 320-1550 / 1-800-952-7687. There is also lots of information at their web site at http://www.prostRcision.com

EDITORIAL COMMENTS FROM AUBREY:

Does Seeding Cause Sterility?

At one of the Seattle conferences, I asked a panel of doctors whether seeding would lead to sterility. One doctor reported that one of his patients, a 70-year-old man who had undergone seeding, was mad as hell. He had assumed that he was sterile because of the seeding, but had just learned that he had impregnated his 27-year-old girl friend.

Everyone is different. In some cases, the seeding does cause sterility. It may also destroy much of the prostate tissue so that there will be very little if any ejaculate, although the man may still enjoy orgasms. The testosterone level should remain the same after seeding, so the libido should still be intact. The amount of sperm manufactured by the testes should remain about the same, but ordinarily, the sperm needs the prostatic and seminal fluids in order to be effective. The prostate may still be able to produce enough of these fluids in some men for fertilization.

It may be possible that the testes could receive a small amount of radiation from the seeds shortly after implantation, but not likely enough to do much damage. However, sperm are constantly dividing and are very vulnerable during the dividing process. It would probably be advisable not to engage in sex for reproductive purposes for at least three or four months after treatment.

COMPLICATIONS

Short term complications were mentioned earlier. There have been several posts from men who have had seed implants. The complication mentioned most often is urgency to urinate, then not being able to. One reason for this is that the prostate has been severely insulted by the needles and the seeds. When a tissue is injured, the first reaction is swelling. The swelling may be so much that it compresses the portion of the urethra that passes through the prostate. This is similar to what sometimes happens in BPH. One of the best treatments for BPH is Hytrin or Cardura. These drugs help to relax the prostate and makes it easier to urinate.

SPREADING RADIOACTIVITY

Someone's wife posted a note on the Internet about possible contamination from her husband's radioactive seeds. Dr. Chris Warner answered:

> "Mary,
>
> Regarding your sleeping arrangements, I am also a physicist. I work at the Walt Disney Memorial Cancer Institute in Orlando, Fl. I will try to give you a technical answer followed by a practical recommendation. The half-life (the time it takes a radioisotope to deliver half of its dose) of I^{125} is 60 days. After 60 days, 2 months, I^{125} delivers half of its dose. Half of the total external exposure to nearby people will be delivered in the first 2 months. For most of the patients that I have measured who have received I^{125} implants, the surface of the patient will measure approx. 0.0015 Rem/hr to 0.002 Rem/hr; at 3 ft from the patient this drops to 0.0001 Rem/hr. As the I^{125} decays over time this dose rate will decrease.
>
> The exposure limit to non-occupationally exposed people is 0.1 Rem per year. If you were to lay on top of your husband 24 hours a day for a year you would receive an exposure of 3.0 Rem in the first year (30 times the recommended limit). Actually, you probably don't spend

24 hours a day with your husband and you probably don't lay on top of him constantly either. You probably spend about 12 hours a day with your husband and on average are about 3 ft away from him. This would result in an exposure of about 0.1 Rem in the first year. As I said earlier, 0.1 Rem is the non-occupationally exposed persons annual limit.

If you were not to sleep with your husband for the first 2 months your exposure would be almost half of this or half of your annual limit. You also have to consider the fact that these annual limits are very conservative, and a few years ago this limit was 0.5 Rem per year. If your husband was to receive a Pd^{103} implant, your exposure would be less because the energy of Pd^{103} is less than that for I^{125}.

With all that said, my personal recommendation would be:

If you are not pregnant and are not planning to be in the near future, I would not recommend changing your sleeping arrangements. The exposure to a spouse of a I^{125} Prostate Implant patient would be at or near the very conservative annual limit.

If you are pregnant or are planning to be in the near future, I would recommend modifying your sleeping arrangements for the first two months for the sake of the embryo. I hope this helps."

Chris Warner, M.S., D.A.B.R. Medical Physicist Walt Disney Memorial Cancer Institute Orlando, Florida

Editorial Note: If one is concerned about his radioactivity after seeding, there are a couple of companies who make lead lined shorts for men. In most cases, they are not necessary. I have not heard of anyone causing any problems to any one else because of their radioactive seeds.

Note that with HDR and external beam radiation (XRT), there is no residual radioactivity.

POST SEEDING PROBLEMS

Here is a letter from Julie about her husband Rudi:

"I'd like to share some problems Rudi is having 2 months after seeding. Mostly, he's fine. He's only missed one day of work. Recall that he's a cop, patrols the streets, arrests people, spends lots of time where urinary urgency wouldn't be an option. He took cardura because he was having trouble starting his stream and keeping it going but the low blood pressure effect didn't work...he said he felt like he was going to faint when he got out of his police car. So he gave it up and is now taking Aleve. He sleeps through most of the night but I think he's still having trouble urinating in one fell swoop.

The really 'bad news'—(everything is relative, when he was contemplating RP, we assumed that intercourse was a thing of the past)—is that when he has an erection and

we have intercourse, it is horribly painful and he feels
like he has to urinate. He says he can't tell the
difference between an orgasm and urinating. Is this a
case of "watch out what you wish for?" Seems like the
wires have gotten crossed somewhere. Comments?" Julie

REASON FOR PAINFUL EJACULATION

Julie mentioned that Rudi had a painful ejaculation. Again, the prostate is a musculo-glandular organ. One of its purposes is to propel the semen out of the penis. To do this it squeezes down and compresses the tissues. Of course, if the gland has not healed from the poking and prodding, then squeezing and compressing the tissues around the seeds will let him know that it is still sore.

COSTS

At the present time, Pd^{103} costs about $50 per seed; I^{125} is a bit less expensive at about $45 per seed. Up to 100 seeds may be used in a procedure.

At one time, there were only a couple of companies who manufactured the seeds. But the seeds have become so popular that it was difficult at times for the companies to supply all that was needed. Several other companies have now entered the field.

FRESHNESS OF SEEDS

Someone asked on the Internet about the "freshness of seeds."
Jennifer Cash, Dr. Dattoli's nurse, made this reply:

> From: <BrachyRN@aol.com>
>
> The Pd-103 seeds are manufactured the day prior to
> scheduled seeding and air shipped to us the evening
> before use. The morning of use, they are loaded and
> recalibrated at that time for dose.
>
> Jennifer>

WHAT HAPPENS TO PROSTATE POST SEEDING

Someone posted a note on the Internet asking what happens to the prostate after it has been seeded.
He wrote:

> "It is my understanding that the way radiation works is
> that it adversely effects all cells, but that normal cells
> are capable of regenerating, whereas cancer cells
> hopefully do not. Now, if the regenerated cells don't
> produce PSA, just how "normal" are they? Could it be
> that the new cells are different in other ways too?"

His note was answered by Jennifer Cash:

> In regards to functioning prostate tissue after seeding:
> In our experience, we have been performing seed
> implants numerous years now, and in the earlier years
> most of our patients treated underwent routine prostate

biopsies between the 1-2 year mark regardless of what their PSA value was. What our pathologists found was residual, viable prostate cells, in addition to radiation fibrosis, and of course, a small subset of patients with residual cancer cells that would be capable of regrowing.

Based on this, we view the effects of radiation therapy of tumor as sterilization rather than complete ablation of normal prostate cells. Also, we have subsequently found that the consistency of the prostate gland resumes to close to normal within 2-3 years post treatment (not remaining like a lump of charcoal as some believe).
Jennifer

Here is another note from Jennifer:

It is very reasonable that after seeding one would expect a PSA nadir of>0 to be normal. We are happy when it drops below the 1.0 value, this has been our best clinical indicator of success. Even though we have a small subset of patients who, when biopsied 1-2 yrs post seeding, had positive biopsies, some of this group went on to have declining PSA's and negative biopsies at later dates. Keep in mind, no treatment has a 100% cure rate!

In reference to the fibrous tissue in the prostate post seeding: Some of the tissue dissolves over time, because, in general, the body does not like scar tissue and, therefore, has the ability to remove some of the scar tissue (just think of other body locations that have had scars and how they diminish over time). Certainly, radiation fibrosis in many patients will persist throughout their life.

We generally see the prostate resume a more normal consistency and size 1-3 years post seeding, and even see a little increase in the size as time passes due to this normalization process and even normal BPH effect with age. Jennifer Cash e-mail: BrachyRN@aol.com. She is a nurse for Michael J. Dattoli, M.D., Cancer Center and Brachytherapy Research Institute

2803 Fruitville Road, Sarasota, Fl 34237 941-957-4926

OTHER BRACHYTHERAPY SITES

There are now hundreds of brachytherapy sites. The web site below lists doctors and brachytherapy sites, by state.

http://www.prostatepointers.org/seedpods/seeddocs.html

Here is a site in London:

The Prostate Cancer Charity

Du Cane Road

London W12 0NN

Tel. 0181 383 8124 (admin), 0181 383 1948 (helpline)

Fax 0181 383 8126

HIGH DOSE RATE TEMPORARY SEEDS

by Drs. Nisar Syed, Ajmel Puthawala & Aubrey Pilgrim

When Andy Grove, CEO of Intel Corporation, was told that he had prostate cancer, he was advised to have surgery. But Andy Grove didn't get to be CEO of a multi-billion dollar company like Intel by blindly accepting advice. He wanted to know firsthand all of the options, benefits, complications and risks. He began to research and study. After doing considerable research, he decided that the best option was the High Dose Rate (HDR) temporary seed implants or brachytherapy. He went to Swedish Hospital Tumor Institute in Seattle and was treated by Dr. Timothy Mate. After his treatment, Andy wrote an article for Fortune Magazine, May 13, 1996. They featured the article and put Andy's photo on the cover. That particular issue of Fortune sold more copies than any in their history. Because of that article, Dr. Mate has been inundated with patients wanting the same type of treatment.

One location that did low dose rate brachytherapy for over 17 years was at the Long Beach Memorial Hospital near Los Angeles. Dr. Nisar Syed and Ajmel Puthawala treated 536 men with low dose rate (LDR) temporary seeds from 1980 to 1997.

Low dose rate (LDR) temporary seeds involved some exposure to the radioactive seeds for both the doctors and nurses. In 1997, the Long Beach Memorial Hospital installed the computers and equipment necessary to perform high dose rate (HDR) treatments. At the beginning of the year 2000, they had treated over 250 men with HDR.

One of the criticisms usually made about brachytherapy is that there is no long-term data. But Dr. Syed has data for 536 patients he has treated with LDR over 17 years. His data is actually better or comparable to surgery for similar stages of tumor. Andy Grove's research showed that the recurrence rate of rising PSA five years after surgery could be as high as 31%. It was as high as 27% for external beam radiation therapy (XRT). For permanent seed implants, it was as low as 19% and for HDR it was as low as 14%.

Of course, recurrence depends to a great extent on initial PSA, stage and Gleason score. Overall, Dr. Syed had a progression free rate of 86% with LDR therapy. Progression free may be higher than 94% if the initial PSA and Gleason score was fairly low. The HDR success rates in the 250 patients treated are even better than the 536 treated with LDR.

The HDR procedure is similar to that of the permanent seed implants in many respects. The prostate size and tumor location is plotted and the treatment dose is generated on a computer. HDR is usually combined with five weeks of external beam therapy and can be used with hormone therapy or as monotherapy depending on initial PSA, tumor stage and its grade.

A couple of very powerful computers are needed for HDR planning and treatment. A lead-lined treatment room is required. A robotic machine to contain and insert the Ir[192] is needed. The machine is under computer control. Fig. 11-2 shows the robotic lead lined housing for the highly radioactive Ir[192] source.

The initial cost of the HDR equipment is much more expensive than that needed for permanent seeds. But the one Ir[192] source can be used several times and may only need to be replaced about three times a year. Considering that permanent seeds may cost from $40 to $50 per seed, over an extended period, the HDR treatment may be less expensive than permanent seeds.

The ultrasound probe is placed in the rectum and a plastic template is held against the perineum. The template has several holes in it to guide the needles. Usually 14 to 16 hollow needles are placed in the prostate under the guidance of the ultrasound probe. Each needle has a short plastic tube attached to the needles. Each plastic tube has a connector so that they can be attached to the tubes from the robotic machine. After the needles are placed, the template is stitched to the perineum. The ultrasound probe is then removed. The needles remain in place in the prostate for the 24 to

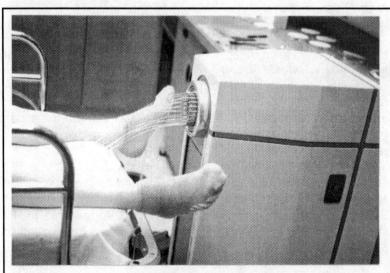

**FIG. 11-2 A HDR Robotic Machine with Patient -
Plastic tubes are used by machine to insert IR-192 source.**

40 hour duration of the treatment. This may be the most uncomfortable part of the whole treatment.

Hollow plastic tubes are attached to the robotic machine that houses the Ir[192] source. See fig. 11-2. A nurse or technician connects the flexible tubes to each needle in the patient. After making sure all the needles are connected, the nurse leaves the lead-lined room and closes the door.

Two video cameras are focused on the patient and the machine. From a separate control room the machine is turned on and controlled by a computer.

There is a single active Ir [192] source in the machine. The source is attached to the end of a thin wire that is inserted into each hollow needle in the patient. The source rotates inside the lead lined machine and inserts the source into each plastic tube in turn. The active source is allowed to dwell for a pre-determined time, then withdrawn and placed into another needle until it has been inserted into each of the needles. The treatment takes about 7 minutes, then the patient is wheeled back to his room, and then 8 to 12 hours later, the same procedure is repeated.

The diameter of the seed source is about 1.1 mm and the length is about 5 mm. (Five mm is a bit less than ¼ inch, so the seed is about the size of a small grain of rice.) The main difference in the HDR source and the permanent seeds is that the HDR source has a much higher amount of radioactivity. Another major difference is that the HDR source is temporarily inserted for a short time under computer control and then withdrawn. One reason for using a machine to insert the source is because of the high amount of radioactivity.

The computer causes the source to be inserted for a previously determined amount of time, depending on the pre-planned dose rate. The machine can be programmed to give a tumor in a certain location of the prostate continuous radiation for a predetermined length of time. Under computer control, the dose rate can be adjusted by having the source dwell for longer or shorter periods of time in certain areas of the prostate. Certain areas such as that around the urethra and the rectal wall can be spared from high doses. A specific dose of radiation can be delivered wherever it is needed.

The pre-planned dosage is given in three or four fractions over 24 to 40 hours depending on the tumor size, PSA and Gleason grade. This doesn't mean that the man will be attached to the machine for this entire length of time. It takes only a few minutes for a fraction of the dose to be delivered. After the fraction is delivered for the planned time, the machine pulls the source back into its lead safe. The Ir[192] radiation in the source lasts for a long time, so it can be re-used several times.

The machine is lead lined so that no radiation escapes when the source is stored inside. Once the source is safely back in the machine, as a precaution, an operator enters the room with a Geiger counter to make sure that there is no radiation still present. The tubes are then disconnected from the man and he is returned to his hospital room to wait for the next fraction. The fractions are given about every 8 to 12 hours. The template and hollow needles will remain attached to the man for the duration of the full treatment time of 24 to 40 hours.

While disconnected from the machine, the man can roll over in bed from side to side, but he is not allowed to get out of bed. Since there is no residual radiation from the treatment, the man can have visitors between the short treatment times.

If necessary, about two weeks after the HDR treatment, the patient may be given a series of external beam radiation therapy (XBRT) to the pelvic region. The amount of radiation received from the temporary seeds may be 2200-2800 centigray (cGY) depending on the initial PSA, stage and Gleason. The follow-up XBRT may be 4000 to 4500 cGy.

They may use hormones with HDR in patients who have locally advanced disease, T2 or T3, high PSA (more than 15) and high grade Gleason score (8, 9 or 10). In these situations they give two to three months of androgen blockade before irradiation, and in some patients who are at a high risk of recurrence and distal metastases, the androgen blockade or hormone treatment may continue for one to three years.

COMPLICATIONS

In the 536 patients that Dr. Syed treated with low dose radiation (LDR), 237 of them said that they had no erectile dysfunction (ED) or impotence before treatment. At a one year follow-up, 71 patients of the 237 (30%) said that they were having ED problems. But as in all radiation treatments, with time, the number of men with ED will increase.

Only six patients treated with LDR had an incontinent problem, four had urethral stricture, or constriction of the urethra that made it difficult to void, and eight had severe proctitis. However, these types of complications are almost completely avoided by using HDR, since it gives the radiation oncologist much better control for radiation dose delivered to critical structures like bladder, urethra and rectum.

Drs. Nisar Syed and Ajmel Puthawala can be reached at the Long Beach Memorial Hospital, Long Beach Radiation Oncology Center
2801 Atlantic Avenue
Long Beach, CA 90801
(562) 933-0300
Fax: (562) 933-0301

OTHER HDR BRACHYTHERAPY SITES

Here is a note posted to the Internet by Joe Armon, armon@ibm.net (Joe Armon):

> For a very simple explanation of the HDR process, check out the site of one of the manufacturers of HDR afterloaders, Nucletron. Go to
>
> http://www.nucletron.com/clin_ap/prostate.htm
>
> There are two HDR treatment centers that have excellent web sites, Tulsa (CTCT) and Oakland (CETMC). They are by no means the only two centers, just the two web sites that give outstanding explanations and illustrations of temporary brachytherapy.
>
> http://www.brachytherapy.com/prost-brachy.html
> http://www.cetmc.com/prostate.html

WHAT SHOULD YOU CHOOSE

Andy Grove said about doctors, "There is no good gatekeeper in this business. Your general internist is not; the field of prostate cancer is a complex and changing specialty. Neither is a urologist; urologists have a natural preference toward surgery, perhaps because urologists are surgeons and surgery is what they know best. Any other treatment is deemed experimental even if it has just as much data associated with it. My review of the data led me to conclude that there are viable alternatives."

Andy Grove strongly recommends that a man should consult the Partin tables to get an idea of his risks. He said, "...I think these tables ought to be posted on the walls of every urologists office. They should be viewed as the point of departure for a prostate cancer patient's bill of rights."

One thing that Andy demonstrated so very well is that it is your body, your disease, and you must take charge. You must do your homework and decide what is best for you. Another point that Andy made was that, even though we only have about ten years of data for this procedure, it looks very good. Even if the cancer recurs at the end of ten years, who knows, maybe by that time we will have found other and better treatments. Maybe by then we will have found the magic bullet.

Andy is still doing well. He is now working with Michael Milken's CaP CURE organization, helping to raise funds for prostate cancer research.

You can reach CaP CURE at 310-458-2873.

HDR is also used to treat cancers of the lung, genitourinary systems, breast, esophagus, pancreas and others.

Chapter Twelve

CRYOSURGERY

By Israel Barken, M.D. <dr@barken.com>

I have been involved from the early beginnings of cryosurgery as it unfolded from an experimental procedure, available in only one state, to a recognized procedure performed in prestigious universities and hospitals all over the U.S. and abroad. We have made a lot of progress. There is a claim being made by the opponents of cryosurgery that there are no long-term results for the procedure. Yet Boney et al (Urology 1982; 19:37–42) reported their results with 229 patients from the mid 1960s with prostatic cancer showing that stage by stage, survival rates compared favorably with those of radical prostatectomy and other modalities that included radiation.

The survival rates of these patients from the mid '60s appeared very promising. The question is then, "Why was cryosurgery abandoned?" The answer is because of the high rate of complications back then. One of the complications was the inadvertent freezing of the rectum, which created rectal fistulas between the prostate, the rectum and the urethra. (A fistula is a connection between two different systems of tubes in the body, in this case between the urinary and the colon tract due to the freezing injury.) In the 1960s, cryosurgery was done blindly without the guidance of ultrasound. At that time the procedure was to make an incision in the perineum and place one probe against the prostate to freeze it.

The issue of efficacy nowadays, since the availability of PSA, is judged differently than in the days prior to PSA. As with any procedure, issues of efficacy and safety have to be taken into account. In the historical cryosurgery, the efficacy, as manifested by similar survival to other procedures, was very good. The safety element of the procedure was poor, which led to the complications. The primary reason for the complications was because of the technique and the primitive equipment that was available at that time. The advances in transrectal ultrasound (TRUS), the development of a computerized machine to control the freezing probes and the development of wires and tubes has enabled us to do precise cryosurgery.

New equipment and technologies are still being developed that include a built-in powerful computer and tanks to hold the gasses used for freezing. The systems may have from four and up to eight freezing probes. Dr. Gary Onik, of Allegheny General Hospital in Pittsburgh, developed the modern protocol. He had gained experience from work on the liver, finding out the signature of freezing on the tissue.

The border of the freezing process is seen as a high dense white line. The ice ball created in the prostate by the freezing can be easily seen with the ultrasound. It can be controlled so that it does not damage the rectum. An initial pilot study was undertaken using five dogs to evaluate the feasibility of using ultrasound to monitor the freezing of the prostate. The animals tolerated the procedure well and there were no complications. (Radiology 1988; 168: 629-631). Soon after this study, Drs. Gary Onik and Jeffrey Cohen in Pittsburgh began the modern version of cryosurgery on the prostate.

ADVANTAGES OF CRYOSURGERY

o Does not require general anesthesia

o No significant blood loss so no need for blood transfusion .

o Procedure takes 2-3 hours.

o Patient may be discharged same day or next day.

o Less expensive than radical prostatectomy or radiation treatments.

o If necessary can repeat the cryosurgery and re-freeze.

o Promising results so far as manifested by rate of negative biopsy and post procedure PSA. Compares favorably to other procedures.

o Little or no incontinence.

o Less traumatic than surgery. Can be performed on men who would not be able to withstand surgery.

o Can be easily performed on obese.

o Procedure can be tailored to preserve potency.

o Cryosurgery has been approved for payment by Medicare and most insurance companies.

DISADVANTAGES OF CRYOSURGERY

o Cryosurgeon has to be very well-versed in ultrasound imaging interpretation.

o Cryosurgeon must be dedicated and experienced in performing this procedure.

o Impotence is comparable to radical prostatectomy in the hands of those who perform an aggressive procedure without regard for preserving potency.

o Equipment and instruments are expensive

o No long-term data.

WHO ARE POTENTIAL CANDIDATES FOR CRYOSURGERY?

o Any patient with localized disease

o Patients with localized disease that are not candidates for radical prostatectomy or radiation treatments.

o Patients with non-localized disease when local control is desirable and patient understands that the intent is not for cure but for debulking and control. Some patients with stage C disease have been treated successfully.

o Patients who are too ill or too old to undergo major, invasive surgery.

o Patients, who psychologically, don't feel comfortable about having major surgery.

o Patients who don't want to take the risk of complications associated with radical prostatectomy such as impotence or incontinence.

o Patients who are psychologically not comfortable with radiation.

Initially, cryosurgery was used primarily to treat those patients who had failed radiation therapy or radiation salvage. Surgery after radiation is not considered a good option because of a high rate of complications. A person can only be safely exposed to a finite dose of radiation. Radiation cannot be repeated. But the disease may still be contained within the prostate in many patients. So cryosurgery seemed to be an ideal solution for these patients. Unfortunately, later experience with this group of patients demonstrated a high rate of complications when cryosurgery is done after radiation. It is very important to choose an experienced cryosurgeon who feels comfortable and knowledgeable taking care of this particular group of patients. This very important point must be disclosed and discussed with patients who have failed radiation.

HOW IS THE PROCEDURE DONE?

Cryosurgery is a procedure by which extreme cold is applied to the tissue. As a result of the low temperature, the tissue is destroyed. Cryosurgery has been done on other tissues of the body such as the liver and the breast. In some cases, such as the liver, an incision is made and the freezing probes are applied directly to the tissue. Prostate cryosurgery is sometimes called percutaneous cryosurgery of the prostate. (Percutaneous means through the skin).

Small probes are inserted through the skin of the perineum into the prostate. The perineum is that area between the scrotum and the anus. An ultrasound probe is placed in the rectum. A picture of the prostate and surrounding tissue is projected on a screen. The freezing probes are almost 1/8 inch in diameter. Several steps are taken before the freezing probes are introduced. By looking at the screen and using the ultrasound guidance, hollow needles are inserted into the prostate.

The prostate is somewhat like an upside down pyramid. The base or largest portion is attached to the bladder. The needles are placed equidistant from each one so that the entire prostate will be covered. Guide-wires are then inserted through these needles and left in place while the needles themselves are retracted. Dilators are gently inserted over the guide wires under visualization on the ultrasound screen. These dilators have a diameter of 3 mm (a little less than 1/8 inch, approximately the size of a drinking straw). They have an external sheath so after the dilator is placed in the appropriate position, the internal portion is removed leaving behind the external sheath. The freezing probes will be inserted through these dilator sheaths.

Some cryosurgeons make an incision so that the dilators will be easier to insert. I don't make any incisions at all but just gently dilate the tracts only. It may not sound important but it avoids the need for stitches. The stitches dissolve by themselves but they can ITCH terribly.

A direct visual examination by a telescopic instrument (cystoscope) ensures that the urethra is normal and will accept a special warmer tube.The interior of the bladder is inspected at the same time that the urethra is checked just to ensure that there is no associated pathology in the bladder. A tiny tube is inserted through the abdominal wall to drain the bladder during the procedure and afterward. The tube (suprapubic tube) is very small and quite comfortable.

Prior to inserting the freezing probes, a special urethral catheter is inserted through the penis into the bladder. This special catheter is similar to a hose that is doubled. Warm fluid is continuously circulated through this catheter to keep the inside of the urethra warm and protected from freezing. (Some have called this catheter a "peter heater.") The cryo probes are inserted into the prostate through the sheaths that were a part of the dilators. These sheaths are then withdrawn so that the metal freezing probes are exposed to the tissue.

The freezing starts as the probes are turned on. Around each probe an ice ball is started. It is well-visualized on the ultrasound screen. The individual ice balls from different probes coalesce to form one large ice ball. The border of the ice ball appears as an intense white line. This white line is carried down the prostate by starting first the upper probes and then starting the lower probes that are closer to the rectum. The rectal wall is also visualized as an intense white line.

The ice ball is allowed to approach the rectal wall. The prostate is very close to the rectal wall. Careful attention must be used to keep the ice ball from freezing the rectum. If the rectum is frozen, it could cause a fistula. A fistula may be very difficult to heal. In order to make sure all of the cancer is killed, the ice ball must come very close to the rectal wall.

Special temperature needles also called "thermocouple needles" are placed in strategic locations in the prostate in order to monitor the temperature during the freezing process. Areas of the prostate may be denser than other areas, especially the tumor areas. The freezing would be different in these areas. By monitoring the temperature with the thermocouples, the freezing can be increased or decreased as needed. The information from the thermocouple needles and the image of the ice ball on the ultrasound screen allows for very close control. Some of the more humorous urological cryosurgeons have called the procedure "ice sculpture." The temperatures will be taken down to –40C or more. Most surgeons will let the tissue thaw and then freeze it again. We define it as the double freeze procedure. The entire procedure, including preparation, may take about two hours.

WHAT TO EXPECT AFTER SURGERY (THE IMMEDIATE POST-OPERATIVE PERIOD)

Genital swelling is very common and of no clinical consequence since the swelling goes down. It usually begins at 2-4 days after the procedure. Discoloration of the scrotum may occur. The swelling and discoloration may disappear in about two weeks. There may be some irritation while voiding. Frequency and urgency are reported in most patients when starting to urinate. How well the patient urinates depends somewhat on the patient's pre-operative capability to urinate. Since the patient has a very small tube draining the bladder through the lower abdomen, it is easy to measure the residual urine in the bladder after urination. The catheter is removed only after patient demonstrates good capability to empty the bladder.

There may be a urethral discharge and some bleeding. A small amount of bleeding may be seen immediately after the procedure staining the protective pad. The patient may pass small fragments of tissue while urinating. This should not cause any significant problem.

POSTOPERATIVE MONITORING

Most cryosurgeons follow the patient with a PSA every 3 months for the first year after the procedure. If there is an indication that the PSA is rising, imaging studies and a possible biopsy may be done. If the patient is part of a protocol study, he may have multiple biopsies at intervals of three months and yearly. There is a tendency to avoid early biopsy in order to avoid creation of a fistula in the immediate post-cryo period.

A new investigational tool to follow patients after cryosurgery is the Spectroscopic MRI performed only at the University of California in SanFrancisco. This test can map the area of question with regard to detecting and differentiating residual benign disease or residual cancer. Whenever possible the author of this article prefers to have this imaging test that provides a "map" to better direct the freezing process. Some cryosurgeons perform multiple biopsies (12–16 samples) in order to get sense of the location and extent of the tumor. This non-invasive Spectroscopic MRI serves as a tool to get the same information achieved by these biopsies without trauma to the patient.

OPTIONS FOR TREATMENT AFTER CRYOSURGERY

Whether cryosurgery followed by hormonal blockade has an advantage has not been proven or disproved. Dr. Horst Zincke did a study showing that hormonal blockade following a radical prostatectomy yielded good results. It makes sense that we can get the same good results with cryosurgery and hormonal blockade. CHT would be especially indicated if the patient's PSA began to rise and systemic disease was suspected or diagnosed.

WHY CRYOSURGERY?

There is a tremendous increase in new cases of prostate cancer every year. The radical prostatectomy has been the "gold standard" of treatment for many years. There has been a lot of disappointment with radical surgery. Surgery is not always curative. "The PSA may start to rise in 50% of patients within five years." (T. Stamey, M.D.: In personal communication). The real percentage of complications from radical prostatectomy may be considerably higher than is being presented in the literature and by practitioners. Impotence and incontinence appears to be much higher than is admitted. For many men, incontinence is a problem that severely affects their quality of life.

Because of the factors mentioned above, there is an increased desire among patients to have a treatment modality that is less invasive and has less morbidity.

THE MAJOR POSTOPERATIVE COMPLICATIONS OF CRYOSURGERY

Urinary rectal fistula, which fortunately happens very rarely and does not happen in the hands of the experienced cryosurgeon, is the most feared complication. This complication occurs also during radical prostatectomy and again rarely in the hands of the experienced surgeon. When a communicating channel opens between the prostate or the bladder and the rectum, it may cause diarrhea due to urine in the rectum and possibly severe infection due to bacteria in the urinary bladder. Fortunately, it is a rare complication and very rare in the hands of the experienced cryosurgeons. It is a condition that can be corrected by local surgery. At times it will close spontaneously by draining the bladder with a catheter.

Urinary incontinence is also an unusual complication in the hands of an experienced cryosurgeon. It is more common in patients that have had prior radiation. There is some degree of mild stress incontinence in the immediate postoperative period.

Urethral sloughing is defined as dead tissue sloughing off from the prostate and being passed during urination. It is possible that this tissue could clog the urethra and prevent the passage of urine. There should be little or no sloughing unless the urethral walls were damaged during the freezing.

Another complication may be the loss of the ability to have an erection, or erectile dysfunction. The penile erection is dependent on the intactness of the neurovascular supply to the penis. Freezing aggressively outside of the prostate gland may injure these nerves that run along the side of the gland. The rate of impotence is similar to the rate due to radical surgery. Dr. Fowler documented an 89% rate of impotence after radical surgery. Dr. Fred Lee reported an impotence rate of 90% at 6 months. The University of San Francisco reported 84% impotence in 6 months. Some small percentage of patients regain erection capability over a longer period of time. In order to make sure that all cancer cells are frozen and killed, many doctors deliberately freeze the neurovascular bundle. Dr. Fred Lee says that if any of his patients are still potent after his treatment, then he has not done it properly.

This issue of preserving the "erection nerves" has to be discussed with the patient prior to the procedure. It is possible to do a "Nerve Sparing Cryo" in patients with a small amount of disease on one side allowing the surgeon to preserve the nerve on the opposite side. Some patients may prefer to do the procedure in two stages in order to try to preserve the nerves and repeat the freezing more aggressively if residual cancer is found later.

Some of the patients may prefer a combination of treatments by doing cryo to destroy the main portion of the cancer and then adopting a modified hormonal approach by using anti-androgens. Lupron and zoladex destroy the libido, but most of the anti-androgens such as flutamide, casodex, nilutamide and proscar usually do not affect the libido.

FACTORS THAT ARE IMPORTANT IN AVOIDING COMPLICATIONS

The training of a cryosurgeon can make a lot of difference. The cryosurgeon's philosophy of treatment and technique is also an important factor that can affect the outcomes. You should look for a doctor who hashad good training and lots of experience.

If the patient has had prior radiation treatment, it predisposes him to a higher risk of rectal/urinary fistula. Having a prior TURP predisposes the patient to urethral sloughing of tissue. The type of equipment can make a difference in outcomes. The newer cryo machine manufactured by EndoCare has built in thermocouple monitoring which provides better control of the freezing process. The type of ultrasound equipment and the urethral warmer used can make a difference. The technique in using the equipment can make a difference. For instance, if the urethral warming catheter is removed prior to the iceball being thawed, this may cause sloughing later.

It is best if you get to know your doctor before treatment and discuss all of these important matters. Ask questions. Talk to some of his patients.

RESULTS OF CRYOSURGERY

Dr. Gary Onik reported negative biopsies in 82.6% of his patients at 3 months following cryosurgery. Dr. Fred Lee found no cancer in 92% of his patients at 3 months. The University of California San Francisco reported that 89% had negative biopsies at 3 months. Dr. Jeff Cohen showed 69% negative biopsy at 21 or more months after the cryo. Overall Fred Lee et al reported negative biopsy rate at 5 years at 82%.

TARGETED ABLATION OF PROSTATE CRYOSURGERY: A NEW AND IMPROVED PROCEDURE

There is a new cryosurgery machine manufactured by EndoCare. Their CryoCare unit uses Argon instead of liquid nitrogen, is smaller and can use 6-8 probes, enabling treatment of larger glands. The new EndoCare machine has a new built in feature—Thermocouples. These are needles that enable us to measure temperature in strategic locations. The panel of this new machine shows a display of temperature. The target is –40 degree Celsius. At this temperature, it was found all living cells die. Hence the name **t**argeted **c**ryo**a**blation of the **p**rostate (**TCAP**). The target refers to target temperature.

TAILORED CRYOSURGERY

If we take it as a given that cryosurgery can achieve the same results as radical prostatectomy, there still remains the question: is it worthwhile to risk the same complications that result from radical prostatectomies. The patient should be a partner in the treatment decision. All patients are different. Some want to make sure every last cancer cell is killed at any cost. Others may want to preserve their potency and accept the risk. The patient must decide how much risk he is willing to accept. Cryosurgery's advantage over surgery is that the procedure is much easier to perform. It is less traumatic. There is no blood loss. There is very short hospitalization of 1–2 days. It heals much quicker, and one can return to work or normal activities almost immediately. These are significant advantages.

The cryosurgical procedure produces good control of local disease, with a good potential for cure. But if we allow complications such as impotence and incontinence to occur at the same rate as radical surgery, then many of the advantages of cryosurgery are lost. I perform cryosurgery after a candid discussion with the patient who has to decide what objectives he feels comfortable with. What does he want to achieve? What can he reasonably expect to achieve? And how much risk is he willing to accept to achieve his objectives? I try to explain to my patients all of the options that he may have such as radical surgery or any of the various types of radiation. I explain the various treatments, the advantages and disadvantages of each. I know that I am a bit biased, but I believe that what I am doing is the best for the patient. But it must be the patient's decision whether he wants to undergo cryosurgery, radical surgery or radiation.

I view cryosurgery as an excellent alternative for patients who have a good understanding of the various procedures. I view cryosurgery mainly as a de-bulking of local tumor (destroying as much as possible the tumor volume). If cure is achieved after first attempt, that is wonderful. I tell my patients, after all the years in practice, I cannot promise to cure everyone. But I tell them that I can avoid most postoperative complications if I am given the freedom to treat fairly non-aggressively. If patient wishes to take the most aggressive approach regardless of complication, I am able to do that for him.

How to correlate the question of efficacy of the procedure compared to the safety of the procedure is very much tailored to the individual. Overall, I don't think that cure is attainable in every case. My motto is: control the disease by conservative treatments but try to do no harm to the patient or detract from his quality of life, and at the same time provide treatments aggressive enough to allow the patient to live out his normal life span. I can't justify the high rate of impotence after cryo that I see in other centers. I think that the patient himself should decide about this very important issue of potency. All men are frightened when diagnosed with prostate cancer. They may panic and act immediately out of fear, only to regret later their loss of their ability to have normal erections because of aggressive treatment.

THE FUTURE

There is further research going on to improve the destruction of the prostate cancer cells by having better mapping to indicate where the location of the cancer is in the prostate gland. If we know exactly where the tumor is, then we can have more success in killing it and perhaps become more selective in our targets of destruction. Spectroscopic MRI may be one of the tools to help us in locating the tumor. Many new developments are in progress. Researchers are working to develop better imaging of the prostate.

Chapter Thirteen

HORMONE TREATMENTS

By Drs. E. David Crawford, Aubrey Pilgrim,
Stephen Strum, Mark Scholz, Bob Leibowitz,
and Eric Small
Contributions by Ralph Valle and
several other PCa Survivors

Drs. Strum and Scholz have written extensively about hormone therapies. Much of this chapter is taken from their writings which are available from Gary Huckabay's Rattler site, www.prostatepointers.org. You can log onto the site and use the search engine to find almost anything you need to know about hormone treatments. If you do not have a computer, by all means you should get one. If you have advanced prostate cancer, a computer can help in your survival.

PSA AND EARLY DETECTION

The PSA test was not generally used before the mid 1980s. Up until 1989, when men were first diagnosed with prostate cancer, 60 to 70 percent of them already had metastatic cancer outside the prostate. Now it is just the opposite. Because of the simple PSA blood test, when now diagnosed, about 75 percent of all prostate cancers are localized within the prostate gland. When still within the prostate gland there are several treatment options. When localized, there is an excellent chance for cure. If the cancer has metastasized outside the prostate, it is systemic. That means that it may be in the entire system. When this happens, there is no way of removing or killing all of the cancer cells. The prognosis is not very good for metastatic cancer. There is no cure, but there are several treatments that can keep the person alive and relatively comfortable for many years. **The answer to cancer is early detection.**

PROSTATE CANCER AND TESTOSTERONE

Most prostate cancer cells must have testosterone and androgenic hormones in order to live and thrive. It is like food to them. Take their food away and many of them will die. So one of the better ways to control prostate cancer, especially if it has metastasized and spread throughout the body, is to control the hormones. Some metastatic cancers may cause a very high PSA, as high as 6000 ng/ml or more. In many cases, combined hormone therapy (CHT) can dramatically reduce the PSA to undetectable levels. There are other metastatic cancers that may have a very low PSA because the cancer cells have mutated to the point that they can no long make PSA.

At one time, very few patients were put on hormonal treatments except those with metastatic prostate cancer. Recently, hormonal therapy is being used extensively as neoadjuvant and adjuvant treatments. (Neoadjuvant means that it is used before the major treatment such as a radical prostatectomy, different types of radiation treatment or cryosurgery. Adjuvant means that it is used in addition to the major treatment.) Some doctors are now using CHT as the primary and only form of treatment. Many of them are having excellent results with CHT as the first line of treatment. It is one of the least invasive treatments designed for a halt in progression, or a remission or even a cure.

WHY CHT WORKS

CHT suppresses the testosterone and other androgens that the cancer cells need in order to grow and survive. Without the hormones, many of the cells starve to death. CHT may cause a vast reduction in the size of a tumor.

In some cases, there may be a few cells that do not depend on the hormones. These are the hormone independent cells. These cells can live and grow without testosterone or androgens. This is called hormone refractory. These are the cancer cells that usually kill a man. This is why it is so important to treat the cancer early before it has a chance to metastasize. Again, the answer to cancer is early detection and treatment.

ACRONYMS

This chapter concerns combined hormone therapy or treatment (CHT). Here are a few acronyms that all mean the same thing:

AAT—Anti-androgen therapy
ADT—Androgen Deprivation Therapy
AHB—Anti Hormone Blockade

AST—Androgen Suppression Therapy

CAA—Complete Androgen Ablation

CAB—Combined Androgen Blockade

CAD—Complete or Combined Androgen Deprivation

CHD—Complete or Combined Hormone Deprivation

CHT—Complete or Combined Hormone Therapy

MAA—Maximum Androgen Ablation

MAB—Maximum Androgen Blockade

NAA—Neoadjuvant Ablation, (hormone therapy before surgery or radiation)

NAB—Neoadjuvant Blockade

TAA—Total Androgen Ablation

TAD—Total Androgen Deprivation

TAS—Total Androgen Suppression

IAD—Intermittent Androgen Deprivation

IAS—Intermittent Androgen Suppression

ICHT—Intermittent Combined Hormone Therapy

IHB—Intermittent Hormone Blockade

IHT—Intermittent Hormone Treatment

We have no doubt that there are many other acronyms that all mean the same thing for this therapy. There must be several people who sit up at night thinking up new acronyms for this single type of treatment. There should be some kind of law or standards for the use of acronyms.

BRAND NAMES AND GENERIC NAMES

Most drugs may have two or more names. There will be a generic name and a brand name. There are two main companies who manufacture the LHRH drugs. TAP Pharmaceuticals makes Leuprolide acetate, brand name Lupron. Zeneca makes Goserlin Acetate, brand name Zoladex. Amgen has a new drug called Abarelix and Alza has developed a one year implant they call Viadur. This drug will be marketed by the Bayer Company.

The antiandrogens are Eulexin, brand name Flutamide made by Schering Corp. and Bicalutamide, brand name Casodex, made by Zeneca. Another anti-androgen that is not used very often in this country is Nilandron, generic name Nilutamide, made by Marion Roussel.

MONOTHERAPY

We have known for some time that both normal prostate cells and cancer cells rely on testosterone to grow. As early as 1893 doctors were doing castration on patients who had obstructions due to BPH. Later it was used for prostate cancer. There was a marked improvement in about 85 percent of the patients.

Castration or orchiectomy is still done today as a treatment. But we now have luteinizing hormone-releasing hormone (LHRH) drugs that can prevent the release of testosterone produced in the testes. Taking the LHRH drugs essentially causes a chemical castration. But, unlike a surgical castration, the chemical castration can be reversed by stopping the drugs. Castration alone, or taking one of the LHRH drugs alone, is called monotherapy or mono hormone treatment. Treatment with one of the antiandrogens may also be called monotherapy.

NORMAL TESTOSTERONE LEVELS

According to an article by Dr. Donald Coffey in Campbell's Urology, the level of testosterone can vary from 300 nanograms per deciliter (ng/dl) up to 1100 ng/dl of blood. That is a very small amount. A nanogram is one billionth of a gram. It takes 28 grams to make one ounce. A deciliter is one tenth of a liter. A liter is 33.8 ounces, so a deciliter is 3.38 ounces. A normal young man will produce a total of about 6 milligrams (mg), or 6 hundredths of a gram, per day. As we get older we produce less testosterone.

According to Dr. Coffey, the level can vary from day to day and even during the day. It is usually highest in the morning. The adrenal glands sit on top of each kidney and produce androgenic hormones in both men and women. The amount of adrenal hormones produced is about 24 mg per day or about four times more than testosterone. These hormones can be transformed into testosterone. But Dr. Coffey says that less than one percent of the circulating testosterone is derived from the adrenals.

SUPPRESSION OF HORMONES SURGICALLY

In the 1940s Dr. Charles Huggins discovered that the androgenic hormones produced by the adrenal glands were quite similar to testosterone. But very little of the androgenic hormones were utilized by the prostate and cancer cells as long as there was plenty of testosterone. However, the prostate and cancer cells are very resourceful. They prefer testosterone, but if it is not present, they will use the androgenic hormones. When testosterone is present, only about 5% of the hormones used by the cancer cells come from the adrenal glands. So even though the testes have been removed, the cancer cells may still get enough hormones from the adrenal glands to thrive. The cancer cells favor the dihydrotestosterone (DHT) form of testosterone. When the testosterone is suppressed, the cancer cells may convert a much larger amount of the adrenal hormones to DHT.

Dr. Charles Huggins studied prostate cancer and hormones for several years. In 1941 he did bilateral orchiectomies on 21 patients who had advanced metastatic prostate cancer. This brought improvement of pain and symptoms in 15 of the 21 men. In 1953 he performed a bilateral adrenalectomy on several patients in addition to orchiectomies. This procedure worked quite well except that at that time it was not possible to replace the vital adrenal hormones that one must have to live. The cancer growth was slowed in most instances, but the patients died due to the lack of the essential and vital adrenal hormones. Today we have several synthetic hormones and drugs that were not available just a few years ago. Dr. Huggins received the Nobel Prize in 1966 for his pioneering work in prostate cancer research.

Among the long-term side effects of castration are hot flashes, osteoporosis, fatigue, loss of muscle mass, anemia and weight gain.

CHEMICAL CASTRATION

There are several drugs that can be used to accomplish a chemical castration. One of the advantages of a chemical castration is that it is reversible. A disadvantage is that the drugs must be taken frequently and are very expensive. Most men will choose the LHRH castration rather than an orchiectomy.

If a man is given estrogen, it will nullify and overcome the effects of testosterone. Conversely, if a woman is given testosterone, it will nullify and overcome the effects of estrogen.

One of the early drugs used for chemical castration was diethylstilbestrol (DES), a synthetic form of estrogen. It is still used in some patients today. It is fairly inexpensive, but it can possibly cause cardiovascular side effects. The original dosage was 5 mg/day. Later studies found that 1 mg/day was just as effective. If DES is used, the patient should be closely monitored for cardiovascular problems such as blood clots.

There are estrogen skin patches that some women have used for hormone replacement after menopause. Some oncologists are using these patches on men as a hormone treatment. Dr. Fernand Premoli of Rosario, Argentina, has been treating a group of HRPC patients for some time with estrogen patches. He has had some very good successes. The estrogenic compounds may cause liver problems when taken orally. The absorption into the bloodstream from the patches helps to avoid some of these problems. But the men still have to be monitored for any cardiovascular or heart problems.

When a man becomes HRPC, it is usually because the androgen receptors (AR) of the cancer cells have become mutated. But the cancer cells may have functioning estrogen receptors (ER). This is why DES and estrogen may work for HRPC. The herbal compound PC-SPES also has an estrogenic effect.

HOW THE CHEMICAL CASTRATION WORKS

A gonadotropin-releasing hormone (GnRH) acts on the pituitary to cause it to release a follicle-stimulating hormone (FSH) and a lutenizing hormone (LH). These hormones occur naturally in the body. They stimulate the testes to produce testosterone. By slightly altering the chemical composition of the natural hormones, we now have Lutenizing Hormone Releasing Hormone (LHRH) drugs that are over 100 times more potent than the naturally occurring hormones. The LHRH drugs stimulate or help in the production of testosterone so are called agonists. See figure 13-1.

The hypothalamus, a small gland in the base of the brain, acts very much like a thermostat. A thermostat may constantly check the temperature in a room, then send a signal to the furnace or air

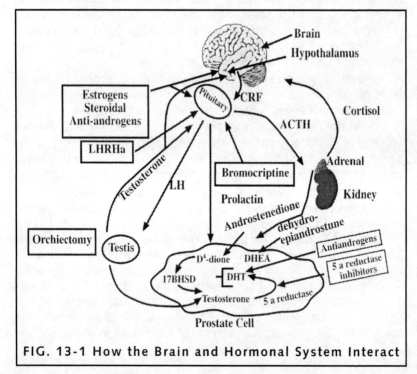

FIG. 13-1 How the Brain and Hormonal System Interact

conditioner to send more heat or cooling. Much like the thermostat, the hypothalamus constantly checks the level of testosterone in the blood stream. The hypothalamus exerts its control over the amount of testosterone in the blood stream by producing a luteinizing hormone-releasing hormone (LHRH). When testosterone falls to a certain low level, the hypothalamus produces LHRH and sends it to the pituitary. The pituitary is a pea-sized master gland in the center of the brain. When the pituitary detects LHRH in the blood from the hypothalamus, it sends a luteinizing hormone (LH) to the testes and tells them to produce more testosterone. When the hypothalamus determines that enough testosterone is present in the blood stream, it stops producing LHRH.

At first the pituitary responds to the abundant synthetic and normal LHRH hormones by producing more and more of the LH hormone. This stimulates the testes to produce more and more testosterone. It may take a few days, or even weeks, but the constant bombardment of the pituitary by the powerful synthetic LHRH agonists finally causes it to become insensitive. The pituitary finally gets to the point where it ignores the LHRH and stops making LH. Without the LH stimulation, the testes stop producing testosterone. These drugs will eventually reduce the testosterone to castrate level and keep it there as long as the patient takes the drugs. Castrate level of testosterone may be 10 to 20 ng/dl.

Zoladex and Lupron are synthetic analogues of the LHRH hormones. These drugs are equivalent to having an orchiectomy. Zeneca did a clinical trial that included 496 men. Of these, 242 were given Zoladex and 254 underwent bilateral orchiectomy. There was no significant difference in survival between the two procedures. If Flutamide, a drug that blocks the uptake of the adrenal hormones, was added to the Zoladex for combined hormone therapy, the average survival rate was 7.3 months longer than patients who had monotherapy.

FLARE

Using the LHRH drugs alone can be the cause of a "Flare Phenomenon." When an LHRH agonist is first started, it paradoxically causes a sharp rise in the pituitary hormone LH. The LH rise stimulates the testicles to increase testosterone production during the first 5-12 days after initiation of the LHRH agonist. This increase in testosterone stimulates prostate cancer cell growth and is termed flare.

WHY IS FLARE PREVENTION IMPORTANT?

In patients with advanced disease and subclinical spinal cord compression, flare can precipitate full cord compression and paralysis.

If there is PC growing close to a nerve root-flare could result in pain in the distribution of that nerve. In patients with PC involving lymph nodes close to the ureters, flare could increase nodal disease and cause early compression of the ureter(s). Obstruction of both ureters could lead to kidney failure. Increasing disease in bony sites often leads to bone pain during times of flare.

Flutamide, Casodex, Nilutamide or any anti-androgen given prior to Lupron or Zoladex can be used to block flare reactions. Other agents like Nizoral, DES or Cyproterone acetate can be used to prevent flare.

It may take one to four weeks after administration of an LHRH agonist to bring the testosterone down to castrate levels. In some cases this may be too long to have to wait. If an immediate effect is needed, a bilateral orchiectomy, Nizoral or Abarelix can be used.

TIME RELEASE DRUGS

The LHRH drugs are in time release formulation. When first developed, the LHRH drugs were given every 28 days. The formulation was then increased to a three month implant, actually 84 days, and now they are available in four month or 112 day formulations. A new LHRH drug implant Viadur, developed by the Alza Corporation, is good for one year.

LHRH ANTAGONISTS

Lupron, Zoladex and Viadur are agonists. These agonists initially stimulate the production of testosterone. Abarelix is an antagonist which stops the production of testosterone immediately. It is quite similar in action to having an orchiectomy. Abarelix is produced by the AMGEN Corporation at www.amgen.com.

ANTIANDROGENIC DRUGS

The adrenal glands produce several androgenic hormones that are similar to testosterone. DHEA and the other androgenic hormones produced by the adrenal glands can be converted to dihydrotestosterone (DHT), the form of testosterone that the prostate cells favor.

Flutamide, Casodex and Nilutamide are synthetic drugs that are similar to the androgenic hormones produced by the adrenal glands. To the cancer cells, these antiandrogens look very much like the real hormones. Cancer cells have a voracious appetite.

When the antiandrogens are present, the hungry cells quickly grab them. The drugs sate their appetite, but the drugs are just slightly different chemically so that they have no nutritive value for the cancer cells. The cancer cells have specific receptors for the adrenal androgens. The receptors might be compared to a lock that will only accept a certain key. When the antiandrogens are present, the cancer cells will let these drugs in. The antiandrogens do not prevent the production of androgens, but if the prostate cell receptors are saturated with the antiandrogens, then very little of the real androgens can enter the cells.

Any one of the antiandrogens can be added to Lupron or Zolodex to form CHT. These drugs can actually stop much of the growth of the prostate cancer.

PROSCAR AND DIHYDROTESTOSTERONE (DHT)

Testosterone and androgenic hormones must be converted to DHT in order for normal prostate and prostate cancer cells to use it. A 5-alpha reductase enzyme is manufactured inside both normal and cancerous prostate cells. The 5-alpha reductase enzyme is necessary for the conversion of testosterone to DHT.

Proscar is a drug that can inhibit the 5-alpha reductase and thus prevent the testosterone from being converted to DHT. Proscar was originally marketed by the Merck Corporation as a treatment for BPH. But many doctors are now using it along with other antiandrogens for prostate cancer. Unlike Lupron and Zoladex, Proscar has few side effects.

Theoretically, Proscar should be all that one needs to combat prostate cancer. It would appear to be an ideal treatment option. The man would still have his testosterone, but the cancer cells would not be able to utilize it. The Government is funding an 18,000 man study to determine if Proscar can prevent prostate cancer. It is a ten-year study and it will be some time before we have the completed data.

ADAPTING TO FLUTAMIDE

The cells in our bodies, including cancer cells, are very adaptable. Dr. Charles Myers says that some of the prostate cancer cells die when their source of testosterone is eliminated. But he says that some cancer cells can mutate and adapt to Flutamide. They use it just as if it were testosterone. If the PSA numbers suddenly start rising after being stable for some time, it may be that the cells have adapted to the Flutamide. If the PSA starts to rise while on Flutamide, often just taking the man off Flutamide will cause a dramatic drop in the PSA. You may see the acronym AAWR, which means antiandrogen withdrawal response. In many cases the PSA will go down and remain down for as long as six months or more.

Some physicians often use Nizoral (generic name Ketoconazole) and Hydrocortisone if the antiandrogens stop being effective.

Nizoral was originally introduced as a drug for toe nail fungus and other fungus conditions. It is also used in shampoos for certain dandruff conditions. It can prevent the production of androgenic hormones. Hydrocortisone must be added to compensate for the vital adrenal functions that we need. Further details regarding the use of Nizoral can be found at www.prostate-cancer.org.

NEOADJUVANT HORMONE THERAPY

Several doctors now start the patient on neoadjuvant hormone therapy (NHT) from three to six months before any major therapy such as a radical prostatectomy (RP) or external beam radiation therapy (XRT). Whenever a RP is done after the patient has been on NHT for some time, some studies indicate that there are fewer instances of extracapsular penetration (ECE) and positive margins. (ECE means that the cancer had penetrated the capsule. Positive margins means that the cancer had penetrated the capsule and had extended beyond the area around the prostate that the surgeon was able to remove). ECE and positive margins generally means that the prognosis is less optimistic.

Neoadjuvant therapy is often used before cryosurgery and brachytherapy. Quite often the prostate may be so large that a large portion is hidden behind the pubic bone and is not accessible for seed implants. At one time they drilled holes in the pubic bone to access these large prostates. They have now found that three to six months on CHT usually reduces the size of the prostate by 40 to 50%. In some cases, they have to be careful not to reduce it so much that there is not enough left for cryosurgery treatment or seed implantation. The normal prostate in a young man should weigh about 21 grams or three-fourths of an ounce. In some older men, BPH along with cancer may cause the prostate to be from 40 grams to over 500 grams. Some prostates have been reduced to as small as 10 or 15 grams on CHT.

For recurrent cancer, combining hormone therapy with other therapies can improve outcomes and survival in many cases.

ADJUVANT THERAPY

Quite often after a radical prostatectomy is done, they may find that the tumor had been under staged. What was thought to be a T1 or T2 (A or B) stage tumor turns out to be a T3 or M+ (C or D) stage. In this case, the doctor may prescribe CHT for a period of time. The patient may stay on CHT for the period, then go off and on CHT intermittently while monitoring his PSA closely.

There have been some studies that indicates that CHT may predispose cancer cells to be more susceptible to radiation kill. If a patient's PSA begins to rise after a radical prostatectomy or radiation, then the treatment of choice should be CHT.

LLOYD NEY AND CHT—A SUCCESS STORY

In 1983 Lloyd Ney was diagnosed with metastatic prostate cancer. A bone scan showed 31 hot spots. One of his doctors told him that he had about three months to live. But Lloyd did not believe the doctor. Lloyd could have chosen to be castrated, but he heard of Dr. Fernand Labrie in Canada who was using some fairly new drugs to counteract the testosterone and the androgenic hormones. Dr. Labrie was pursuing the same line of attack that Dr. Huggins had tried when he removed the adrenals. The difference was that now there was no need to remove the adrenals because chemical drugs were available that could counteract the testosterone and adrenal hormones. Dr. Labrie called his treatments combined hormone therapy or CHT.

Many doctors did not accept the findings of Dr. Labrie. They pointed out that the adrenals contribute a very small amount of testosterone. They were convinced that monotherapy was all that was needed. One of the problems was that it takes years to prove something like this. To do a proper test, several men of the same age, with the same type and stage of cancer, should be randomized into two groups. One group would get the monotherapy and a placebo and the other group would get monotherapy plus an antiandrogen. Then you would have to wait until the men died to determine which was the better treatment. In some cases, this might take up to ten years or more.

Since the combined hormone treatment didn't cause any additional damage or side effects, why not go ahead and use it. Later studies were made by the Schering Company, the manufacturer of Eulexin or Flutamide. Their studies indicated that CHT had a distinct advantage over monotherapy.

Lloyd went from Grand Rapids, Michigan over to Canada, met with Dr. Labrie and began taking combined hormone treatments. Lloyd felt better almost immediately. He wanted all prostate cancer patients to be aware of the hormone treatments and that CHT should be available to all patients. He began publishing a newsletter, called the Cancer Communication. He formed a nonprofit organization called **Patient Advocates for Advanced Cancer Treatment (PAACT).** Lloyd began petitioning the FDA and Congress to approve the hormone treatments in this country.

After seeing the success of the treatments in Canada and other countries, many doctors in this country began using the hormone treatments even though they were not FDA approved. It wasn't until 1989 that the FDA finally approved the treatments. A lot of the credit should go to Lloyd Ney for his persistence. Lloyd accumulated a list of over 30,000 prostate cancer survivors who received his newsletter. He spoke personally on the telephone with many of these men, giving them advice and counsel and hope. Thousands of these men will tell you that they owe their very life to Lloyd Ney. Lloyd died on August 19, 1998, 15 years after being told that he had only three months to live. He was 78 years old.

Almost up until the day he died, Lloyd answered the phone and talked with men who had questions about their cancer treatments. Lloyd said that he got a phone call one day and the man asked if the hormone treatments would affect his sex life. Lloyd said, "I don't know. How old are you?" The man said "94." It just goes to show that you are never too old.

Though Lloyd is gone, the PAACT organization survives. Call them at (616) 453-1477 and they will answer your questions, send you a packet of information about prostate cancer and put you on their mailing list for the Cancer Communication Newsletter. They don't ask for any contribution of any kind. But it does take money to run a foundation such as PAACT. Any money donated may be deductible from your income taxes.

DR. FRED LEE: PROSTATE CANCER SURVIVOR

In 1983, Dr. Fred Lee was 51 years old. He was a successful radiologist, a loving husband, and the father of five children. After watching a manufacturer's demonstration of an experimental transrectal ultrasound machine, he scheduled a demonstration test on himself. At that time, transrectal ultrasound was so new that no one was able to read the images. However, the salesperson commented that Dr. Lee's images looked different from what was normally seen. This led to the discovery that Dr. Lee had prostate cancer.

X-ray tests did not reveal evidence of cancer spread, and Dr. Lee was hopeful of a cure using radioactive seed implant. At that time, the procedure was performed by making an abdominal incision and manually placing the radioactive seeds directly into the prostate. Several days later, Dr. Lee discovered that his lymph nodes were found to contain metastatic prostate cancer. Because of the positive lymph nodes, Dr. Lee underwent an additional course of external beam irradiation to the whole pelvic region. Additionally, he started taking Emcyt, which he continues to take to this very day. Emcyt is a combination drug consisting of estrogen and nitrogen mustard. It is often used as a chemotherapy.

Unfortunately, in 1986 a repeat biopsy confirmed persistence of his prostate cancer. He received an additional course of external beam to his prostate as well as four courses of hyperthermia. Dr. Lee has been rebiopsied three times since then with no evidence of cancer and his PSA remains extremely low.

Dr. Lee learned that only 50% of men with his stage of disease live for 5 years and only 10% live for 10 years. Dr. Lee decided to dedicate the time he had left to optimize the detection and treatment of prostate cancer. Dr. Lee's work defined what prostate cancer looked like on transrectal ultrasound. This led to its widespread acceptance as the preferred method of diagnosing prostate cancer. He was the co-chairman of the American Cancer Societies National Prostate Cancer Detection Project, a multi-institutional study involving over 2000 men. He has written or co-authored over 75 publications, has been visiting professor at numerous institutions, and has made countless presentations. Currently, Dr. Lee is the Director of the Crittenton Hospital Prostate Cancer Center in Rochester Hills, Michigan. Dr. Lee has specialized in doing cryosurgery. Since his arrival, over 700 cryoablative procedures have been performed at Crittenton Hospital.

Dr. Lee is now 68 years old and still going strong at Crittenton Hospital, 248-652-5611.

JEROME MAN, ANOTHER SUCCESS STORY

Here is an e-mail from Jerry that I received in early 1997. "When I was diagnosed in 1988, I telephoned Dr. Labrie in Canada for Flutamide which I obtained during a visit to Dr. Strum in Culver City. I had been examined by doctors at the City of Hope and by Dr. Israel Barken (he should be designated as a National Treasure) in San Diego. I am now seeing a wonderful Oncologist/Urologist, Dr. Paul Brower, in Laguna Hills, California. Until September 1995, I was employed full time as a federal agent, and retired at that time. I am 73 years old, no metastasis. Current medications include Proscar, Casodex, and lots of pumpkin seeds (a good source of zinc) and some garlic (selenium). I monitor my urine flow rate DAILY using a calibrated container, and determine the volume for a 30 second period of time. This tells me the amount of restriction of the urethra caused by the prostate or tumor. My highest PSA was 5,953 ng/ml and was last measured at 377 ng/ml."

I, Aubrey, talked with Jerry and invited him to come to one of our support group meetings. He wasn't sure he could make it. He was taking some college courses, had homework to do and had several other projects going. One other thing that kept him busy was being president of one of the largest computer user groups in the Los Angeles area.

Unfortunately, Jerry died on Aug. 24, 1998, over ten years after being diagnosed with a PSA of 5,953. He was 75 years old.

LARRY PARKS, AN ENIGMA

Below is the digest of Larry Parks. He had a beginning PSA of 408. With a PSA that high, there is usually lymph node involvement and/or bone metastases. But despite several tests, no evidence of metastases could be found. A biopsy showed a Gleason score of 7.

Larry began CHT and his PSA came down to as little as 0.6, but then it went back up to as high as 39. He tried several different drugs and External Beam Radiation. At the time of this writing in 2001 his PSA is 1.76.

Larry wrote:

> <I have been concerned about posting my results because, as you are well aware, this disease does not affect all sufferers equally.
>
> Fondest Regards,
>
> Larry>

He is so right about the statement above. Again, the first rule when it comes to cancer is that there are no rules.

THERE ARE NO PANACEAS

CHT worked well for Lloyd Ney, Jerry Man and thousands of other men. Dr. Labrie has been completely vindicated for his early stand on CHT. He is honored and respected by the entire medical community. As Chief Oncologist at Laval University, in Canada, he conducts studies and research on prostate cancer. We cannot ever forget that we are all different and our cancers are also different.

Dr. Labrie has said several times that we could eliminate advanced prostate cancer and eliminate the untimely deaths of thousands of men each year. All it would take is early detection. **The answer to cancer is early detection**.

CHT COMPARED TO OTHER TREATMENTS

While there are some undesirable side effects of CHT, they are fairly mild compared to some of the side effects of the other treatments. One of the major side effects is the loss of libido. A radical prostatectomy may leave a man with an intact libido, but unable to have a normal erection. Once hormone treatments are interrupted, the libido and potency may return. If the nerves that enable erections have been severed during a prostatectomy, then the man will never be able to have a normal erection. Another side effect of a RP is that many men are rendered incontinent. Incontinence may be more of a problem than impotence. The CHT does not cause incontinence. A radical prostatectomy is major surgery. It may be quite traumatic for some men, especially older ones. CHT is much less traumatic. When compared to radiation, cryosurgery and other forms of treatments, CHT also seems to be as good as or better in many respects.

CHT3 AS PRIMARY TREATMENT FOR CLINICALLY LOCALIZED AND LOCALLY ADVANCED DISEASE

Dr. Bob Leibowitz is an oncologist who practices in the Los Angeles area. He strongly believes in conservative treatment. He treats all of his patients with combined hormone therapy, but he goes a step further and adds Proscar, or Finasteride, to the LHRH and antiandrogens for triple blockade or CHT3. He started treating some of his patients as early as 1990 with this protocol. He now has a group of 98 patients that are being followed. Each have completed 13 months of triple hormone blockade for clinically localized and locally advanced disease. His story was published in *The Oncologist*, April 2001.

Here are some vital statistics:

Patients	AGE	Mean Age	
15	50-59	67.1	
50	60-69		
29	70-79		
4	80 and over		
Patients	bPSA	Mean PSA	Mean PSA 2 1/2 yrs
10	<4	13.55	Off Treatment is 1.4
45	4-10		
24	11-20		
19	20		

Lowest bPSA = 0.39 Highest bPSA =100

Patients	Gleason	Mean Gleason
2	4	6.55
13	5	
35	6	
35	7	
5	8	
6	9	
2	10	

Note: bPSA is beginning PSA before treatment.

All men were treated with Lupron or Zoladex LHRH agonists. In addition to the LHRH agonists, the men took either Flutamide 125mg, 2 capsules every 8 hours, or 3 Casodex 50mg tablets at one time daily. (Note that the standard dose of Casodex is usually a single 50 mg tablet per day). The men also took 5mg of Proscar

(Finasteride) per day. During treatment, the PSA levels became undetectable in all patients within three or four months.

Dr. Leibowitz keeps his patients on this protocol for 13 months. He then has them continue with 5mg of Proscar each day for maintenance. As of December 1999, he had 60 patients who had been off treatment for at least 12 months and some patients had been off for as long as 73 months. Average time off treatment for this group is 2 1/2 years. The mean PSA is 1.4 and is stable.

The testosterone levels of 37 men were measured before treatment. The testosterone ranged from a low of 123 to a high of 635.During the 13 months of treatment, the testosterone fell to castrate level. But after treatment the testosterone production returned. For all men off treatment for at least one year, the testosterone levels ranged from 11 and up to 893 with a mean of 403. The libido usually returned to normal along with normal sexual functions.

Dr. Bob Leibowitz can be reached at 310-229-3555, fax 310-229-3554, e-mail beewell@earthlink.net

The CHT3 treatment is one of the least invasive of all treatments. The hot flashes, no libido and other unpleasant side effects usually last for one year only or the duration of treatment. The side effects of some of the other treatments last for the rest of your life. One other big advantage is that, after treatment, the man still has his prostate. He has no incontinence and can still have normal erections, orgasms, and even ejaculations.

Another advantage of this protocol is that it is one of the least expensive. The drug costs will be approximately $12,000 for the 13 months. Of course the office visit costs would have to be added. The cost of the Proscar needed for maintenance would cost about $1000 per year.

Still another advantage is that there would be no hospitalization or outpatient care or cost. There would be no time lost from work or recuperation.

Some men have gone on CHT and stayed on it for years even though their PSA became undetectable after just a few months. When these men finally go off CHT, it often takes a very long time for their testosterone production to become normal again. In some men it never recovers. Also many of these men never regain their libido and lost muscle mass. If a patient has an undetectable PSA for at least a year, it would seem better to go on intermittent treatment. This may help prevent the cells from adapting to the CHT. If the PSA starts rising while off treatment, the patient can always go back on therapy.

TIMING OF TREATMENT

Like most things in life, there is a cost, or downside, to CHT. There are several side effects that severely affect one's quality of life (QOL). One of the most unhappy side effects for many men is a loss of libido. The enjoyment of sex depends on the libido and without testosterone, there is no libido.

Without testosterone, the patient may feel tired and fatigued. He may have a loss of muscle mass. Men produce both testosterone and a small amount of estrogen from the adrenals. Without the testosterone, the estrogen exerts a greater influence on the man. His breasts may become very tender and sore and may also become quite enlarged. And he may put on weight.

A very famous surgeon and a few other doctors believe that, because of the psychological and sexual side effects of hormonal treatment, it should be delayed until progression of disease. However, if hormonal therapy is delayed until the tumor burden becomes massive, a proportionally larger number of androgen-independent cells may persist after hormonal therapy and be much more difficult to control. We think that the preponderance of evidence supports early hormone treatment rather than late therapy.

Dr. E. David Crawford, Dr. E. Messing and several others did a study titled, "Immediate Hormonal Therapy vs. Observation for Node Positive Prostate Cancer Following Radical Prostatectomy and Pelvic Lymphadenectomy." The study was published in a leading peer review journal and was also presented at the 1999 AUA Convention.

Between 1988 and 1992, 98 men with node positive (N+) prostate cancer (PC) who had undergone radical prostatectomy and pelvic lymphadenectomy (RP+PL) were randomized to receive bilateral orchiectomy or goserelin acetate (patient's choice) vs observation (Obs) with hormonal therapy (HT) administered upon progression.

At mean follow-up of 7.2 years, 6 of 46 men in the Early Hormone Treatment (EHT) arm had died, 2 from PC. In the Obs arm, 18 of 52 had died, 16 due to PC. Four of 46 EHT men have progressed/recurred (including the 2 who died of PC) and 5 have experienced biochemical failure (PSA 0.4) only. In the Obs arm, 29 have progressed/recurred (including 16 who died of PCa), and 10 had a rising PSA or biochemical failure. Thus, 18.8% EHT vs. 75% Obs patients have failed.

In men who had positive lymph nodes during a radical prostatectomy, early hormonal treatment (EHT) significantly prolonged survival compared with observation and delayed HT. This is the first demonstration of a survival advantage for EHT in a randomized prospective clinical trial in which only the effects of HT on the disease itself (and not on assisting other treatments such as radiotherapy) have been tested. Extension of these results to even earlier disease settings merits further investigation.

There are thousands of men who gladly endure the unpleasant side effects of hormone treatments because the alternative is much worse.

PROSCAR AND FLUTAMIDE OR CASODEX AS PRIMARY TREATMENT

Several men are using Proscar and high dose Casodex (150mg/day) or Flutamide as a primary treatment. This does not cause a suppression of the testosterone. It does not cause hot flashes, loss of muscle mass or most of the other unpleasant side effects of CHT. It may cause a loss of libido in a small number of men.

The man can go on this protocol and closely monitor the PSA. If it starts to rise, then he can always go to the other more radical options. This is one of the least invasive of all treatments.

COSTS OF HORMONE TREATMENTS

One of the easiest and least expensive ways to deprive the prostate cancer of testosterone is to simply remove the testicles or castration. The Greek term for the testicle is *orchis*. A more euphemistic term for castration is orchiectomy or orchidectomy (orchid plus *ectomy* which means excision or removal). Later a flower was discovered that had a root or bulb system that looked a bit like a testicle. Since most flowers and plants are given Greek and Latin names, it was called an orchid.

An orchiectomy is fairly simple and may have a one-time cost of less than $2000. Even after an orchiectomy, a man may still have to take one of the antiandrogens. An orchiectomy plus an antiandrogen and LHRH plus anti-androgen are both equivalent to combined hormone therapies.

The International Pharmacy at www.internationalpharmacy.com lists thousands of drugs and their prices. If you are buying drugs, it is a great place to do some comparison price shopping. Here are some prices for CHT drugs:

Lupron depot (28 day) 7.5 mg	$680.67
Lupron depot (84 day) 22.5 mg	$2042.03
Lupron depot (112 day) 30 mg	$2722.71
Zoladex (syringe 28 day) 3.6 mg	$516.99
Zoladex (syringe 84 day) 10.8 mg	$1550.98

Casodex (30 tablets) 50 mg	$380.41
Casodex (100 tablets) 50 mg	$1268.05
Nilutamide (90 tablets) 50 mg	$291.82

They did not list Flutamide. A local drugstore offers it at a senior discount rate of $60 for 30 125 mg capsules. The normal dose is two capsules every 8 hours, or six per day. This would be $12 per day or $360 per month.

The doctor visit for the injection will add to the cost of Lupron or Zoladex. Medicare and most insurance companies pay for the drug and the cost for the doctor to give the injection. But Flutamide, Casodex and Nilutamide are prescription drugs. The doctor gives the patient a prescription and he fills it at a pharmacy. At the present time, Medicare does not pay for these drugs, but many of the insurance companies do. Hopefully, Medicare may pay for some of this cost in the future. The total cost for CHT may be $750 and up to $1500 or more per month or up to $18,000 or more per year. If the man lives for ten years, it could cost over $180,000 for drugs. Both surgical castration and chemical castration have the same side effects. Both procedures eliminate the libido, cause hot flashes, loss of muscle mass, and osteoporosis.

Since orchiectomy and CHT procedures are equivalent, you can understand why HMOs, Medicare and some doctors urge the men to undergo surgical castration. (If cost is a major consideration, castration can be accomplished for much less than $2000. For years, farmers and ranchers have been putting a rubber band around the testicles of male animals to castrate them. The rubber band cuts of the blood circulation and in a short time the testicles just fall off. We can only hope that Medicare, HMOs and insurance companies don't find out about the rubber band).

If chemical castration is equivalent to surgical castration, why don't more men choose the less expensive orchiectomy? There are several reasons why men choose LHRH agonists. First and foremost, the chemical castration is reversible.

They hope that someday soon, a magic bullet will be found that can eliminate their cancer and they will be whole again. There is also the hope that their cancer will go into remission. It does happen in a small number of cases. Some of them feel that it is bad enough to have to give up sex due to the hormone treatments. But undergoing castration removes just about the last vestige of their manhood or any hope of recovery.

Holding on to their testicles is so important to some men that they do it with both hands. Many of them feel that a man has to have testicles in order to be a man. Some have argued that there are probably other hormones and substances produced by the testes besides testosterone. So why not keep them if the drugs will do the job. Once the testes are removed, they are gone forever. We keep hoping that a new cure may be found someday that will make prostatectomies and castrations unnecessary.

INTERMITTENT CHT

After a period of time on CHT, the PSA of many patients goes to zero or to a very low level and remains steady. In some patients the PSA becomes undetectable in a very short time. In others it may take several months. The length of time from beginning CHT to undetectable can be a fairly good prognosis of the course of the disease.

If the PSA goes to undetectable and stays there for a year or so, some doctors believe that it is beneficial to take the patient off hormones for a period of time. One reason for going off the hormones is so that the cancer cells do not become adapted to the hormones and learn to live with them. The cells in our bodies, including cancer cells, can learn to adapt to and live with almost anything. Our ability to adapt is one of the reasons for evolution.

If a person is placed on antibiotics for an extended period of time, the bacteria may learn to adapt and evolve to the point that the antibiotics are no longer effective. It is quite possible that the cancer cells do the same thing when a man stays on CHT for a very long time. We know that they often learn to actually thrive on some of the antiandrogens. Some of the cells actually die when the antiandrogens are withdrawn, called the antiandrogen withdrawal response (AAWR).

Going off CHT is beneficial to the patient's quality of life. Without the hormone treatments, the patient's testosterone level will usually return along with his libido. The resumption of testosterone levels will also make the patient feel stronger and feel better.

Still another reason to go intermittent is that you save the cost of the drugs. Many men go on CHT and continue on it for years, even though their PSA is undetectable. These men are at risk for the cancer cells to become refractory. Another reason to go intermittent is that millions of dollars could be saved if all the men whose PSA has gone to undetectable and stayed there for at least a year went intermittent.

While off the hormone therapy, the PSA level is closely monitored and if it begins to rise, the patient resumes the CHT treatments. Several men are trying intermittent therapy. Some men go off all drugs. Others go off the Lupron or Zoladex and take an antiandrogen such as Flutamide or Casodex along with Proscar. This allows them to regain their libido and overcome the constant fatigue.

DR. STRUM'S INTERMITTENT THERAPY PROTOCOL

We believe in a prolonged exposure to CHB with nondetectable PSA reached and sustained for 12 months. In our study population the average time OFF therapy after the above is achieved has been 20 months with the longest time off 48 months. If the patient's PSA begins to rise, when it gets to about 5 ng/ml we restart them on CHB.

Our initial period is 12 months of NONDETECTABLE PSA (NDPSA). We follow this, upon reinitiation of CHB with the same approach: 12 months of non-detectable PSA. So far no one has failed this approach. We have been doing it for over 7 years.

Dr. Strum has published the results of his studies. It is the largest trial of patients on IAD with the longest followup. Some patients have been off treatment for over 8 years with a flat PSA.

His article on Intermittent Hormone Blockade was published in the February 2000 issue of *The Oncologist*. You can view the abstract and the full lengtharticle by going to:

http://theoncologist.alphamedpress.org/cgi/content/abstract/5/1/45

Drs. Strum and Scholz have a web site or a HOMEPAGE at :

www.prostate-cancer.org (see their papers, software, resources, etc) for other resources such as the PCAB (Prostate Cancer Address Book) with phone numbers, addresses and e-mail of outstanding people in the world of PC.

PC PAPERS AND COMPUTER SOFTWARE: go to their web site to download these without charge. Also see CLINICAL RESEARCH PUBLICATIONS in peer-reviewed journals written by Strum & Scholz.

Web: www.prostate-cancer.org

A FEW PATIENTS WHO OPTED FOR IAS

W.J.KENNEY wjkenney@prodigy.net

> I was diagnosed with a PSA of 49.8 in 1992. I was treated with RP and then with External Radiation Therapy. Have been on CHT on and off since then. Off for as long as 24 months sometimes. Now over 8 years since diagnosis.

BILL CANNON CarlsbadBill@prodigy.net (Bill Cannon)

> I had an RP in 1992, started CHT in February, 1995 with a PSA of 18—and stopped in July, 1995. PSA WAS 0.1 in August, 0.64 in November.Have been on and off several times. As of August 2000, I continue on Intermittent.

GEORGE McCALL mccalls@earthlink.net

I had a PSA of 14.7 July 7, 1994, Gleason was 1+2=3. Chose to watch and wait. April 11/95 PSA was 20, May 16, PSA 27. Went on CHT in June, 1995 as an initial treatment with a PSA of 27. Stopped CHT in September 95 with PSA of 0.3. May 96 PSA was 6.3, August 9.0, November PSA was 8.3 after 13 months off CHT. October, 1997...PSA increased to 17.4. At 77 years old, went to Dr. Gordon Grado in Scottsdale, AZand had Seed Implants. Minor side effects; Last PSA 0.3 in June 1999. October 1999—The only lingering side effects I experience are decreased libido, frequent and slightly burning urination. I will be 80 years old in a couple of months, so I feel very fortunate to have fared this well with this terrible disease.

Editorial Note: Note that George's Gleason was 1+2=3 with a PSA of 14.7. He had an enlarged prostate, probably due to BPH which can produce PSA. But his PSA continued to rise and was almost doubled from 14.7 on July 7, 1994 to 27 on May 16, 1995. No doubt this indicated an aggressive cancer. The Gleason Score of 1+2=3 was probably an error.

CHARLES CLAUSEN cclausen@magick.net

Born 7/37, 1/94 PSA 9.9, Gleason 3+4, bone scan neg, cT2c or cT3a (acid phosphatase 0.4, normal on assay = 0 to 0.8)

3/94 RP at UCSF, pT3aN1 (4 cu. cm. volume of tumor, extensive perineural and vascular invasion, extensive extracapsular extension in right posterior lobe with focal extension to surgical margin, sv & vas neg, 0.4 cm. met in 1 of 10 lymph nodes)

Since his RP in Jan. 1994, Charles has been on and off CHT three times. His on cycles have been for as long as 8 months, his off periods have been as long as one year.

Charles uses the ultrasensitive PSA tests. He is quite knowledgeable about it and wrote the article on ultrasensitive PSA in Chapter 6. He spends a lot of time on the Internet answering questions.

DON SWIRNOW swirnow@qwestinternet.net

DOB=7/20/32, Dx=8/92, PSA=21, Gleason of 7, aborted RP in 9/92 due to one bad lymph node. CHT started in 10/92 giving PSA of 1.0 in 12/92, less than 0.1 from 4/93 thru 3/96 when CHT stopped. Five needle biopsy in 3/96 all negative for PC. PSA on 6/4/96 was 0.1 and 0.39 on 9/4/96. Started Proscar (5mg 2x/day) on 8/1/96. MRI/MRS in October showed no detectable cancer inprostate or seminal vesicles or lymphs. On 11/5/96 reduced proscar to 5mg per day due to gynecomastia.

He has been off CHT for as long as 18 months or more before starting again.

"I guess I should have been dead years ago". ☺—Don

Editorial note: Don has spent a lot time learning about prostate cancer. He devotes a lot of time to the Internet answering questions and helping others.

ORCHIECTOMY AND IAS

Here is an Internet post from Dr. David Michener who had an orchiectomy:

> "Subj: [PP] Testosterone replacement clearing house
>
> From: bermich@EARTHLINK.NET (david michener)
>
> I am seven years into hormone blockade beginning with one year of Lupron followed by orchiectomy with gratifying PSA response but considerable aggravation from side effects. After following the positive reports from intermittent blockade, I have been working with my oncologist to simulate intermittent by getting testosterone supplements.
>
> After eight months of monthly IM testosterone enanthate I have been very pleased with the results. The PSA has gradually approached 5 which may be a good cut-off point. In any case, I am aware that there are others out there post—orchiectomy who are looking for something better. I know that both Dr. Strum and Dr. Leibowitz have such patients and I assume that there are others.
>
> I would be glad to hear from any of you and to provide a point for collection of our pooled data. Your identification can remain anonymous, if you wish, and I would be happy to distribute whatever information we obtain. Specifically, it will be helpful to know what routes of administration work (I know that transdermal gel and oral DHEA have been tried) and what cut-off points have been determined.
>
> Certainly, the responses of circulating testosterone and PSA levels will be of interest. Let me know of any interest and I'll be glad to share.
>
> David P. Michener, M.D. MPH"

There are other men who have had an orchiectomy who are experimenting with testosterone replacement.

Here is some information from Dr. Bob Leibowitz:

> "I am now treating men with testosterone replacement therapy. All were previously surgically castrated. All had undetectable PSA's; hence, they were hormone sensitive. They wanted to be on intermittent androgen blockade, but lacked the necessary equipment to produce their own testosterone.
>
> When I reviewed the information available on why it is generally felt that testosterone replacement is contraindicated in a man with metastatic prostate cancer, I concluded that this statement is accurate for any man with hormone resistant or hormone refractory disease. If, however, you are still hormone sensitive, then testosterone may not be harmful (my opinion for these

men only). Do not apply this rationale to your situation; this has the potential to worsen your prostate cancer and hasten complications and/or even death.

If testosterone were harmful for all men with prostate cancer, then no one should ever be allowed to stop hormone blockade, since stopping blockade almost always results in your testosterone rising to pre-hormone blockade levels. Intermittent hormone blockade would not be allowed if all doctors believed that testosterone is harmful to all men with prostate cancer.

One patient has been on testosterone replacement for about one and one-half years. His PSA is about 0.26 and not rising. He feels much better; much stronger; and hits his golf ball 25 yards further than pre-testosterone days.

Another patient has been treated with testosterone for over one year and has a stable PSA of 0.4 (by a different PSA assay). He also feels much better and has improved his golf game.

One other patient has only been on treatment a few months. He still has an undetectable PSA.

I must stress that any decision to consider testosterone replacement therapy must be made on an individual basis, and I urge you to never try it if you are hormone resistant at all. Your PSA will rise if you do."

Several of the men being treated by Dr. Leibowitz belong to the various support groups in the Los Angeles area. Many of them are personal friends of co-author Aubrey. Here is a letter that was received from one of them:

"Dear Aubrey,

The success of my treatment should give encouragement and optimism to others. It all started with a radical in 1988, stage C, Gleason 3+4, positive margins. Remember this was before PSA. I had 6700 rads of broad beam radiation after the surgery. In 1993, I had a rising PSA that was doubling every 2 weeks. My choice at that time was to have an orchiectomy. This is a choice that most would not make, but I think it was a good decision. Later I added Casodex and Proscar to my regimen. My PSA has been undetectable ever since. It is quite likely that the triple hormone blockade therapy might have been equally effective, but I did not know about it at that time.

To counteract some of the detrimental side effects of the CHT, I have now been off Casodex for 1 1/2 years and only on Proscar maintenance. After many months of study and analysis, I have now begun using a rub-on gel form of testosterone supplementation. My testosterone level has risen to 125 while my PSA is still undetectable.

This last 11 years has caused shock, anxiety and despair. But it has also caused excitement, acceptance and a sense of accomplishment. I am winning the battle.

James, E. Ahrens, Ph.D."

OSTEOPOROSIS

Osteoporosis is one of the symptoms of Androgen Deprivation Syndrome. Osteoporosis is quite common in post-menopausal women. One reason is due to the lack of estrogen. (The prefix *osteo* is from the Greek for bone, as you might guess, *porosis* means porous). Osteoporosis is also one of the major side effects of long term CHT. I wrote about my friend, Jerry Man, earlier. He had had a PSA of 5,953 in 1988. He was on CHT for ten years. He claims to have lost almost six inches in height. Some of that was due to his "dowager's hump," which is often seen in older women.

Osteoporosis is a serious problem for men on long-term CHT. Many doctors do not assign enough significance to it. Bones are easily broken and may take a very long time to heal. Fractures of the spine, hip and wrist are common.

There is some information about osteoporosis at this Merck web site: http://www.merck.com/product/usa/fosamax/cns/dosing/dosing.html.

This site talks primarily about women, but osteoporosis affects men on CHT in the same way.

TREATMENT FOR OSTEOPOROSIS

Bisphonates are one of the treatment options. Fosamax (Alendronate Sodium) is often used. FOSAMAX˚ (alendronate sodium) is an aminobisphosphonate that acts as a specific inhibitor of osteo-clast-mediated bone resorption. Bisphosphonates are synthetic analogs of pyrophosphate that bind to the hydroxyapatite found in bone.

PC-SPES

Several men are taking PC-SPES as a primary treatment or as a treatment for recurrent prostate cancer. In most men, it lowers the PSA and appears to control the cancer in the same manner as CHT. However, there is no long-term data as to its efficacy. Dr. Eric Small of the University of California at San Francisco is doing one of the few studies of the herbal compound.The article below is taken from Dr. Small's study.

PC-SPES (PC stands for prostate cancer, SPES is Latin for hope), a dietary supplement, is a combination of eight Chinese herbs that have long been used in Asia to treat various medical conditions. It is commercially available at health food stores as an over-the-counter supplement for the treatment of prostate cancer; however, due to the possible side effects, it is recommended that PC-SPES be taken under the supervision of a doctor.

UCSF has treated 70 patients with PC-SPES. Half had hormone-sensitive disease (had never before received hormonal therapy), and half had received hormones and had developed hormone resistant prostate cancer.

In brief, our findings suggest that patients who have never been treated with hormones will virtually all have a significant response to PC-SPES. One hundred percent of patients had a decline in their PSA, and 56% of patients achieved an undetectable PSA. However, this was felt to be due to the hormonal effects of the drug, which resulted in a dramatic decline in the male hormone testosterone in over 80% of patients. Ninety-two percent of these patients developed breast tenderness or swelling, symptoms that are very reminiscent of treatment with hormonal therapy. Thus, we feel that at a minimum, this product has hormonal effects, at least in patients with hormone sensitive disease.

However, we were surprised that in hormone resistant prostate cancer patients (patients who had already received hormones, and despite hormones had developed growth of their cancer) approximately 60% of them had a significant PSA decline (defined as a decline of more than 50%, lasting for at least a month). Furthermore, in those patients who were tested, some patients had improvement in bone scans and other measures of disease. Thus, we believe that PC-SPES probably has some activity in patients with hormone resistant prostate cancer.

It is important to note that for both groups (both hormone sensitive and hormone resistant) we do not know how long PC-SPES will work, and what, if any, long-term complications exist. Short-term complications have been reasonably mild. The retail cost of PC-SPES through the manufacturer, Botanic Lab, is $108 per bottle of 60 capsules. At 9 capsules per day, the cost for a month of therapy is $453.00. Unfortunately, at this time there are no insurance companies, HMOs, Medicare or other third party payers that pay for the use of PC-SPES. This may change over time, but for now the cost of PC-SPES unfortunately must be borne by the patient.

A supply of PC-SPES may be obtained from Botanic Lab, 2900 B Saturn Street, Brea, CA 92821. The phone number to order the drug is 800-242-5555. Botanic Lab's web site is http://www.botaniclab.com. PC-SPES does not require a prescription, but it is advisable to take it under the supervision of a doctor.

PC-SPES ONLINE SUPPORT GROUP

There is another PC-SPES web site at www.PC-SPES.com. They have a lot of up to date information about the product. They also have an on-line support group that you can join. This group is made up primarily of patients who are taking PC-SPES. You can e-mail them with questions or suggestions.

WHY PC-SPES MAY BE EFFECTIVE

PC-SPES has a phytoestrogenic component. Prostate cells have androgen receptors (AR) and estrogen receptors (ER). Even those cancer cells that have become hormone refractory may still have estrogen receptors so they will respond to estrogen therapy. Estrogen patches and DES may provide an equivalent therapy at a much lower cost.

TREATMENTS FOR HORMONE REFRACTORY PCA

There are several chemotherapy treatments that can be used if the patient has become hormone refractory (HRPC). One of the more promising treatments seems to be taxotere. We will talk about that and other treatments in the next chapter.

Chapter Fourteen
CHEMOTHERAPY
Drs. E. David Crawford, Aubrey Pilgrim, Stephen Strum, Israel Barken, Bob Leibowitz and Contributions from Several Survivors

INTRODUCTION

Chemotherapy is the use of drugs that hopefully will kill more cancer cells than normal cells. It is used primarily for advanced metastatic disease. This is a chapter that is challenging to write because until recently there were very few positive chemotherapy drugs and treatments that we could write about. This is not to say that you should be discouraged and give up hope. There is hope and there are many new drugs and protocols that are being investigated. Just hang in there.

We mentioned it before, but if you do not have a computer, by any and all means, get one. It can help you enormously. Computers are fairly inexpensive today. Even if you have to give up going to the opera a couple of times, or out to a fancy dinner every other night, use the money to buy a computer. There are thousands and thousands of web sites that offer tons of information. Use the computer to search the web sites. You can use www.google.com, www.yahoo.com, www.excite.com, www.lycos.com or any of several other search engines. Then type in whatever you want to search for and you will be amazed at the number of sites that have the information you are seeking. Much of the information is revised and updated often.

PROSTATE CANCER AND BREAST CANCER

You can search the Internet for prostate cancer and will see many sites, but if you search for breast cancer you will be presented with about ten times as many as for prostate cancer. You can search for prostate cancer AND chemotherapy and you will see very few sites.

Do the same for breast cancer AND chemotherapy, and, again, you will see about ten times more sites.

You will also see that the chemotherapy for breast cancer has more positive results than treatments for prostate cancer. Fortunately, many of the chemotherapy drugs used for breast cancer can also be used for prostate cancer. Unfortunately, they don't always work as well on men as on women.

One of the reasons we see so much more about breast cancer is because they have raised much more money for more research. We men should be ashamed of ourselves because we have not done more to help ourselves.

HORMONE REFRACTORY PC (HRPC)

Co-author E. David Crawford, writing in *UROLOGY* 54-51-52 1999, has an optimistic view of successful HRPC treatments:

> "Although severing the grip of hormone refractory prostate cancer (HRPC) still eludes us, there is reason to be optimistic that we may soon witness a change. Several chemotherapeutic and biologic agents (taxanes, estramustine, antisense oligo-nucleotides) have been evaluated in phase I and phase II clinical trials with encouraging outcomes; phase III trials are currently being developed. A phase III trial of the chemotherapeutic regimen of combined mitoxantrone and prednisone has shown improvements in outcomes.
>
> "More importantly, however, are the cases of complete or partial response that are being observed with these newer treatments. Data emerging for the taxanes, alone and in combination with estramustine, have renewed interest in chemotherapy for HRPC. Equally promising is the confirmation that newly recognized cellular mechanisms may represent exploitable vulnerabilities in the disease process.
>
> A rationale for early treatment is that within prostatic tumor masses, as with many other cancers, genetic heterogeneity of the malignant cells increases with tumor enlargement. This heterogeneity makes it less likely that any form of treatment can affect a durable response. Thus, controlling cellular proliferation with earlier treatment might minimize the appearance of genetic diversity within tumors."

You have seen the word heterogeneity mentioned several times. Heterogeneity means that several different cells appear such as those which become hormone independent. Homogeneity would mean that the cells are all the same.

The treatments that we have for early stage prostate cancer, in the majority of cases, may either cure it or hold it in check for several years. But in some cases, in spite of all we do, the cancer may break through and the PSA will start to rise. Combined Hormone Therapy (CHT) is usually our first line of defense after a surgical or radiation treatment failure. The CHT may work for some-time, but some patients eventually develop hormone refractory prostate cancer (HRPC). HRPC may also be called Androgen Independent PC (AIPC). Advanced PC may not be the same thing. Advanced PC can be cancer that is outside the prostate, but it may still be responding to CHT.

We don't know why some men become refractory to CHT. Some believe that there are hormone independent cells from the very beginning of the cancer. When the patient then goes on hormone therapy, the dependent cells are killed off, leaving only the cells that do not depend on hormones to survive and proliferate. It is these hormone independent cells are that eventually kills the patient.

Others believe that the hormone independent cells are due to cell mutations while on hormone therapy. They believe that the longer one waits before going on hormone therapy, the longer he has freedom from the AIPC. No one knows for sure what the answer is. Some very prominent doctors recommend that hormone therapy should not begin until there are symptoms. Symptoms are usually due to bone pain. At this stage, usually there is widespread metastases.

WHEN TO START TREATMENT

Logically, it would seem that the sooner one began treatment with hormones, the less tumor burden and the more control that can be exerted. We believe that CHT should be instituted early and so do a lot of other doctors.

When the PSA continues to rise and no longer responds to maximum androgen blockade (MAB) or CHT, there are several chemotherapeutic drugs and protocols that can be instituted. The taxanes, paclitaxel and docetaxel seem to offer a lot of hope. Taxol and taxotere are the active ingredients in these drugs. They have worked very well for breast cancer.

HARRY PINCHOT—A HRPC SURVIVOR

Harry Pinchot is an example of a survivor with HRPC. He is a young man who became hormone refractory and had some chemo treatments. He was 54 years old on 9/21/94 when he had his first PSA of 16.9 and a negative biopsy. On March 30, 1995 his PSA was 31.2 and another biopsy confirmed cancer. He began CHT but his PSA never went to undetectable. It went to its lowest on 8/02/95 when his PSA was 0.2 using the Immulite ultrasensitive test. He decided to go on injections of Velban, oral Emcyt and radiation. His PSA went down to .01 on 9/26/95. He stopped his CHT. But then seven months later, the PSA started creeping up again.

On 5/09/96 his PSA was 3.17. He resumed CHT and added thalidomide to his regimen. On 11/12/96 faced with a rising PAP and an inability to reduce his PSA to non-detectable, he added PC-SPES at 6 capsules. His PSA on 12/26/96 was .003. On 4/11/97 he stopped lupron and Eulexin and on 5/13/98 thalidomide was stopped. As of March 2001, with a dose of 12 capsules of PC-SPES and 10 mg of proscar per day, his PSA is .003 using the ultra sensitive test.

Harry is an active member of several of the Los Angeles area support groups where there are several other survivors much like him. He also works with Dr. Strum's Prostate Cancer Research Institute (PCRI).

WHEN CHT FAILS

One of the drugs used by many oncologists when the patient stops responding to CHT is Ketoconazole, brand name Nizoral. It is usually given with aminoglutehimide.

Dr. Stephen Strum is an oncologist. He answers questions from patients on an Internet site called P2P, (Physician to Patient). You can send e-mail to: p2p@www.prostatepointers.org. Here is part of one of his responses to a patient:

> <My PSA rose again, this time to 14.0 which has totally frightened me. I have a few questions as follows:
>
> 1) do you still recommend nizoral when the PSA jumped from 10 to 14 in one week?>

> "Nizoral or Ketoconazole is an excellent agent for both androgen dependent PC and androgen independent PC. It can be used in combination with other agents due to it being synergistic with drugs such as velban and adriamycin, and perhaps Taxotere."

> <2)An oncologist recommends starting chemotherapy with taxotere. Do you agree and do you recommend a particular protocol (a few options seem to have been presented.)>

> "We are using weekly taxotere at 25 mg/M^2 of body surface area. This amounts to about 50 mg average dose for most men. This is well tolerated. We often combine the taxotere with another agent such as carboplatin or cytoxan and 5 Fluoracil".

Note that the dosage listed above is "25 mg/M^2 of body surface area." We are all different. The M^2 means per meter of body surface squared. A man who weighed 150 pounds would not be given the same dose as a man who weighed 300 pounds.

When and if the patient stops responding to one protocol, there are several other drugs. Here are just a few that are often used for chemotherapy:

Adriamycin, Cyclophosphamide, Estramustine, 5-Fluorouracil, Gemcitabine, Mitomycin-c, Navelbine, Nitrogen Mustard, Taxol, Taxotere, Trimetrexate, Vinblastine, Mitoguazone, Doxurubicin, Epirubicin, Mitoxantrone (Novantrone), Strontium 89 (Metastron), Samarium 153 (Quadramet).

Here are a few drugs that are sometimes used in combination:

Cisplatin plus Doxorubicin, Cisplatinum plus Etoposide, Methotrexate plus Buserlin, Estramustine plus Doxorubicin, Estramustine plus Etoposide, Estramustine plus Navelbine, Estramustine plus Taxol, Estramustine plus Vinblastine, Navelbine plus Taxol.

This is not a complete listing of chemo drugs. Many new ones are being investigated and developed.

Dr. Mark Scholz, an oncologist who works with Dr. Stephen Strum had this to say on the Internet to a patient:

> The most active chemo agent in prostate cancer is Taxotere. It is much more active than Novantrone. If it is ultimately proven that you have metastatic prostate cancer to the liver then I recommend that you take taxotere 25 mg/m2 every week. The side effects are mild and there is at least a 50% chance that it will be beneficial.
>
> Mark Scholz M.D.

HOW THE DRUGS ARE GIVEN

Chemotherapy may be given by different methods. Most often it is given by injection into a vein or intravenously. It may also be injected intramuscularly or under the skin (subcutaneously). It can also be given orally or by mouth, (the prescription may say PO which means Per Os—Os means mouth).

Sometimes the drugs are diluted into a large bag of liquid and given via a "drip" into a vein in your arm or hand. In these cases, a fine tube will be inserted into the vein and taped securely to your arm.

Another way of giving intravenous chemotherapy is via a fine plastic tube (called a central line) put into a vein in the chest. Unlike the cannula used for the vein in an arm, a central line is inserted after one has been given a general or local anesthetic. Once it is in place, the central line is either stitched or taped firmly to the chest to prevent it from being pulled out of the vein. It can remain in the vein for many months. This will reduce the need for needles when given the intravenous chemotherapy. Blood for testing can also be drawn through this line.

Chemotherapy may also be given by using infusion pumps. The pumps are portable and come in various types. They can be used to give a controlled amount of drugs into the bloodstream over a period of time.

SOME OF THE SIDE EFFECTS

We are all different and have different diseases. We may not all react the same way to a treatment. But here are some general side effects that one may expect on some of the chemotherapy drugs: nausea and vomiting, fatigue, hair thinning and loss, diarrhea and constipation, mouth and gum problems (stomatitis), skin and nail problems, sexual problems, low blood cell counts, gynecomastia, hot flashes, weight loss, weakness, and several other unpleasant side effects.

Many people are able to carry on with their normal life while on chemotherapy. It is important that you do not become depressed or lie in bed and vegetate. Do everything that you possibly can to improve your quality of life. If possible, travel and do all the things you have always wanted to do.

If you have pain, do not hesitate to ask your doctor for pain relief. Don't worry about becoming addicted to pain killers. You may even be able to have an occasional drink of alcohol. Just check with your doctor and make sure that alcohol does not interfere with your medications.

You can find out more about chemotherapy by going to the site below: http://www.bethisraelny.org/healthinfo/chemotherapy/index.html

CLINICAL TRIALS

We discuss abstracts later in this chapter. Many of the abstracts are summaries of clinical trials that have been done. There are all kinds of clinical trials. Every drug approved by the FDA has had to go through some sort of trial. Here we are discussing clinical trials for cancers.

Charles J. McDonald, M.D. is National President of the American Cancer Society. In a letter to the U.S. News and World Report, 11/29/99, he says that "...one out of every three women will get cancer in their lifetime and one out of every two men will get it in their lifetime. Currently, only 55 percent of cancer patients are cured. Participating in a clinical trial offers the best and most appropriate treatment for many patients. These are innovative treatments. In the absence of standard treatment, therapy through a clinical trial may be the only way to help a patient. Remember, what was "investigational" a few years ago is often the standard treatment today. Countless Americans are alive today because they participated in a cancer clinical trial."

SHOULD I JOIN A CLINICAL TRIAL?

Here is an article by Israel Barken, MD (619-287-8866)

This article is written for the patient who is about to say, "I'm ready to join a study." Some patients reach this stage because they have exhausted all other avenues of treatment. They are dying, and they have nothing to risk. Therefore, any gain at all is a benefit.

The patient needs to approach joining a study in the most egoistic manner. The most important question is why should I join the study? What is in it for me?

A little background about the nature of clinical studies is helpful here in understanding where the clinical trial you are about to enter has its roots. There are some parts to the process before a trial enters human work. First, the search for new treatments starts in the laboratory where the idea of a drug is tried in test tubes or glass plates. If it is a proposed cancer drug, tumor cells may be grown in culture and the drug is tried there. This is called an "*in vitro*" study. If there is success in this stage, the research goes on to the next phase. If the idea is found to be valid in test tubes, then the treatment is tried on animals. Two factors are tested on the animals: the efficacy of the drug and the safety of the drug. It is absolutely critical for the reader to understand this one point: **what works in test tubes or on animals may not work at all on humans.**Therefore, I believe that it is important for the patient to have a disclosure of the initial basic research results and to consult your doctor to help you understand these results.

It is standard practice in Phase I to recruit a small number of patients, usually three patients at each dose level. The dose is raised until either the patient gets sick or the desired result is achieved. Once that level is achieved, six or more patients are then treated with the same level to make sure it is a safe dose. The main question here is: **How safe is the drug and at what dose?** The highest dose that can be tolerated is the focus of the experiment here.

In Phase II, the attention is shifted from safety to efficacy. (Note that only about 70% of studies make it from Phase I to Phase II.)

The dose has been determined in Phase I. Now, the highest safe dose is given to 14 patients. If none of these patients respond, the drug is considered worthless. If one patient responds then a total of 30-40 patients are treated. One of the advantages of this phase is that usually there is no randomization of the patients.

Phase III (Note that only about 33% of all trials enter Phase III investigation):

In this phase the new treatment is compared to the standard treatment. Phase III is initiated only after the treatment has shown some promise in Phases I and II. Phase III includes a large number of patients in multi-centers. Patients are usually randomized to receive the standard treatment or the new drug.

In a Phase IV study a known proven medication approved by the FDA from previous studies is being checked for a different indication or different dose setting. Data is collected and compared to established treatments.

Patients with very advanced disease and no available treatments may get a drug which is not yet approved and is not available on the market. Under *"compassionate use,"* the drug can be given on an individual basis. For example, thalidomide is available to be given to individual patients who have run out of available treatments through a special arrangement with the FDA.

In summary, only 30% of Phase III studies are submitted to the FDA for approval. Of these, only 20% are eventually approved by the FDA. It may take a company 2-10 years to complete the studies on Phases I, II, and III. It may take the FDA 3-20 years to approve the final product. (No wonder that drugs cost so much.)

In looking at an individual clinical trial, here's what you need to know:

Each study is carried out according to a strict action plan. This action plan is known as the *"protocol."* The protocol explains what is done during the period of the study. Each study has to be approved by an *"Institutional Review Board"* or IRB. The IRB is a committee of health professionals, members of the community like clergymen, lawyers and patient advocates. They are responsible for the study being appropriate and avoiding unethical risks.

Selection criteria for studies is a key element in the clinical trial. This is described in the protocol. The eligibility criteria are important for the researchers. They will seek to create groups of similar patients. *You may not qualify under their criteria.* Before traveling to an institution for the purpose of joining a study, have your doctor make the initial connection with the researchers and make sure you qualify. Two main areas for refusing patients to a study are:

1. Patient must have good organ function. These include liver function, kidney function, adequate number and function of blood components.
2. Have had no prior treatment which would make evaluation of the study difficult.

You will receive a document called "*Informed Consent*" which basically explains the study and your rights as a patient. You will be asked to sign this document so take the time to ask questions of the researchers, study it and understand it before signing.

What are the possible benefits you can derive from joining a study? There are many. You may receive treatment in a center of excellence and have a very tightly controlled environment in which you can follow your disease through many tests that otherwise would not have been done.

If the treatment in the study is effective you may be one of the first ones to enjoy a good result. This is especially true with the more advanced phased studies. You may have the cost of your care covered by funds provided for the study. By being part of the study you may feel good by doing something altruistic for society.

There are also some possible drawbacks to be aware of when joining a study. They are:

New treatments under study are not always better than standard treatments.

You may suffer from side effects that even the researchers did not suspect.

You do not have any control over which arm of the study you are assigned to. Neither does your referring physician. You may get a placebo in certain instances.

You may incur some costs for your medical care that may not be covered by your insurance. Be alert and carefully check the financial rules of the study.

What are your rights as a patient contemplating joining a study?

You and only you have the right to choose a study versus standard existing treatments. It is wise to involve your own doctor in this decision.

You have the right to leave the study at any time without any need to give any explanation.

You have a right to have your privacy protected.

You must be given an Informed Consent document to read and sign. All the facts of the study should be given to you. This should include explanations about the treatment, tests, risks and benefits and financial coverage.

Any new information while you are on the study should be given to you. You have the right to ask the doctors how the study is going with other patients and you should get honest answers.

CancerBACUP has an excellent web site with lots of information about clinical trials, sexuality and most other aspects of what you can expect while on chemotherapy. Visit their web site at: http://www.cancerbacup.org.uk/info/chemotherapy.htm

NATIONAL CANCER INSTITUTE (NCI)

The National Cancer Institute is a part of the National Institute of Health, a branch of government. It is an excellent resource and provides lots of information. Many of the items are in blue text. This means that they are automatically linked to a page or another URL (Uniform Resource Locator) site that has more information about that item. Just click on the blue text and it will take you to the new area. There is usually one or two arrows at the top left corner of the page. If you click on the left pointing one, it will take you back to the last page you were on. Click on the right pointing one will take you to the next page.

CANCER INFORMATION SERVICE (CIS)

Provides accurate, up-to-date information on cancer to patients and their families, health professionals, and the general public. Information specialists translate the latest scientific information into understandable language and respond in English, Spanish, or on TTY equipment.
   Toll-free: 1-800-4-CANCER (1-800-422-6237) *TTY:* 1-800-332-8615.

CLINICAL STUDIES SUPPORT CENTER

Provides information for patients and physicians seeking information on the National Cancer Institute clinical studies at the Clinical Center in Bethesda, Maryland. Available Monday-Friday, 9 am-5 pm EST.
   Toll-free: 1-888-NCI-1937

E-MAIL—CANCERMAIL

Includes NCI information about cancer treatment, screening, prevention, and supportive care. To obtain a contents list, send e-mail to cancermail@icicc.nci.nih.gov with the word "help" in the body of your message.

FAX—CANCERFAX®

   Includes NCI information about cancer treatment, screening, prevention, and supportive care.

To obtain a contents list, dial **301-402-5874** from a fax machine hand set and follow the recorded instructions.

CLINICAL TRIALS

NCI's trials database, PDQ® (see User's Guide for search tips)
New! Conducting Trials: Resources for Health Professionals

EDUCATIONAL RESOURCES

Taking Part in Clinical Trials: What Cancer Patients Need to Know
Taking Part in Clinical Trials: Cancer Prevention Studies
Cancer Facts—brief summaries of subjects related to clinical trials, provided by the Cancer Information Service
Prostate, Lung, Colorectal & Ovarian Cancer Screening Trial— this site provides information about participation in the PLCO trial, a large-scale effort to determine whether screening healthy people for these cancers can result in early detection and lower death rates.

For information about clinical trials taking place at the NCI/National Institutes of Health campus in Bethesda, Maryland, see the Bethesda Campus Clinical Trials site.

Bulletin: High Priority Trials Seeking Patients

Certificates of Confidentiality: Background Information and Application Procedures—Certificates of Confidentiality allow researchers to avoid the involuntary release of any portion of research records containing information that could be used to identify study participants.

GENERAL CANCER INFORMATION

CancerNet—CancerNet contains material for health professionals, patients, and the public, including information from PDQ® about cancer treatment, screening, prevention, supportive care, a searchable listing of clinical trials, and CANCERLIT®, a bibliographic database.

For a complete introduction to many types of cancer, see the What You Need to Know series.

Cancer Information Service—a national information and education network.

Cancer Facts—a collection of fact sheets that address a variety of cancer topics.

Questions about Cancer—This page offers Frequently Asked Questions and information about how to ask your own questions electronically or by telephone.

WEB PAGE

The Main NCI Page at http://www.nci.nih.gov/ is NCI's primary web site. It contains information about the Institute and its programs. It has a wealth of information.

Rex is a site that includes news, upcoming events, educational materials, and publications for Patients, Public, and Mass Media.

SOME HRPC ABSTRACTS

The Internet is a fantastic way to find out about chemotherapy and treatments. If you visit the American Society of Clinical Oncologists (ASCO) web site at www.asco.org and do a search for Hormone Refractory Prostate Cancer, you will find several abstracts.

You will find several abstracts at the American Urological Association (AUA) web site. You can search their web site at www.auanet.org.

The web sites are updated frequently. They can let you know of new research and discoveries. By all means you should have a computer that will allow you to take advantage of these resources.

Many of the abstracts are about Docetaxel, Estramustine/ Etoposide, SU101, Paclitaxel, Estramustineand Carboplatin.

THE PROTOCOL OF DR. BOB LEIBOWITZ (310-229-3555)

I strongly recommend applying our most effective systemic treatment "up front." I believe it is a major mistake to "save your best weapon for last." The best time to attack prostate cancer is the first time. If it is time to consider chemotherapy, use it now, and use the most effective treatment; essentially with no exceptions.

Do not wait and allow prostate cancer cells the time to mutate and become more aggressive. We know cancer cells undergo additional, molecular biological hits (mutations) that make them more resistant to treatment. These additional hits or mutations apply not only to hormone sensitive cells, but also hormone resistant. Hormone resistant cells continue to undergo additional molecular biological changes and mutate to ever more resistant cells. Hit them hardest early.

I give Taxotere-based chemotherapy, either E.T./C.D. or T/E/D for about 16 weeks. What follows is the treatment program I usually recommend to my patients. I cannot recommend this to anyone who is not my patient. That decision can only be made by you and your oncologist.

T/E/D PROTOCOL:

I began using what I called the T/E/D protocol about one and one-half years ago. This consists of weekly low dose Taxotere, along with Emcyt two days a week and Decadron two days a week. I treat three weeks in a row, then one week off.

At times, I have added a fourth medicine, carboplatinum (once a week, intravenous), and I call the four drug program E.T./C.D. (the initials of each of the four medicines Emcyt, Taxotere, Carboplatinum and Decadron).

All of the men are also on once a month Aredia and daily Proscar. For the E.T./C.D. protocol, I simply add carboplatinum, 100 to 125 mg/m2 (total dose 200 mg or 250 mg rounded off) each week. So far, I have not seen any extra toxicity by adding carboplatinum, except for some mild reversible hair loss. I have administered several hundred doses of carboplatinum to date, and this observation is most impressive and accurate. I predict that the E.T./C.D. program will ultimately be shown to be even more effective than T/E/D. I have begun to recommend using prophylactic Coumadin, a blood thinner to prevent blood clots (thrombophlebitis). There is a risk of blood clots from Taxotere/Emcyt or Taxol/Emcyt.

These two Taxotere-based chemotherapy regimens debulk cancer much more effectively, in my opinion, than Nizoral-type, alternate hormone blocking regimens, and this puts you in remission. Then use Nizoral or aminoglutethimide as maintenance therapy, to maintain your remission.

I also urge liberal use of Aredia. I often utilize Aredia plus E.T./C.D. or T/E/D as my first treatment for men with hormone resistant or hormone refractory prostate cancer.

SUMMARY

There are studies that appear to show an improvement in survival in some men treated with chemotherapy. Trials are ongoing to evaluate chemotherapy that is given early in the disease, before the patients becomes hormone refractory.

A number of drugs are showing promise including combinations of drugs. Mitoxandrone and Prednisone have been shown to improve quality of life. The combinations of Taxotere and Estramustine Phosphate have yielded some significant PSA responses.

Gene therapy, antiangiogenesis drugs, drugs that block the cell's signal that inhibit the cell from aging (anti-sense bcl-2) are among some of the more exciting therapies being evaluated.

Lots of research and clinical trials are being done. Eventually they will find a cure for cancer or at least find a way to keep it from killing you.

We hope that you can find a treatment that will work for you.

A SAD NOTE

In the first edition of this book, in this chapter, we wrote about Scott Barker, Len Snyder and Russ Ingram. They all put up a good fight, but lost the battle. This book is dedicated to them and the other thousands of men who have also lost the battle.

Chapter Fifteen

INCONTINENCE

By Drs. Barton Wachs and Aubrey Pilgrim

INTRODUCTION

Incontinence is a major problem. About 17 million people, mostly women have this embarrassing problem. It also affects many men who have had treatments for prostate problems.

In a search of the Internet there were nearly 100 sites that offer products and treatment advice for incontinence. This may surprise you, but here is one of the sites:

4th Quarter, 1999—November has been declared "<u>Incontinence Awareness Month</u>," and perhaps no other non-fatal condition is so deserving of such a designation. Incontinence (involuntary loss of urine) is common; an estimated 17 million Americans, the majority women, experience it; incontinence is expensive, the annual U.S. price tag approaching $20 billion, and for the afflicted individual, incontinence can be socially devastating.

<u>http://usrf.org/news/incontinence.html</u>

We list the rest of the web sites at the end of this chapter. The first part of this chapter is by Aubrey Pilgrim, the second part is by Barton Wachs, MD. His father has advanced prostate cancer, so he is very much interested in prostate cancer. He set up a support group at the Long Beach Memorial Hospital. Dr. Wachs mother and father usually attend the monthly meetings. He has been very generous of his time in helping people.

TYPES OF INCONTINENCE

There are five basic types of urinary incontinence:

Stress Incontinence

The involuntary loss of urine associated with increased pressure on the bladder such as coughing, sneezing, laughing, bending, or lifting.

Urge Incontinence

The compelling need to urinate and the inability to stop leakage long enough to reach a toilet.

Mixed Incontinence

The most common form of urinary incontinence. Inappropriate bladder contractions and weakened sphincter muscles usually cause this type of incontinence. This type is a combination of the symptoms for both stress and urge incontinence.

Overflow Incontinence

This form of incontinence results in continued leakage of urine because the bladder is full beyond capacity.

Functional Incontinence

Factors outside the lower urinary tract, such as deficits in physical and/or cognitive function cause this form of incontinence.

PROSTATE CANCER SURGERY AND INCONTINENCE

One of the major problems men have after prostate surgery is incontinence. A quality of life (QOL) study done by UCLA found that for those men who were incontinent, it was more of a problem than impotence. Some statistics say that most men are able to regain control by the end of 24 months in about 98% of cases. Other estimates place the number of men who are incontinent to some degree as high as 10% especially during the first year or so after a radical prostatectomy. A few have incontinence problems that may be longterm and severe. Some may have to use several pads or adult diapers per day.

Generally, the more procedures a doctor has done, the greater his expertise andthe less complications with incontinence and impotence.

SPHINCTERS

A sphincter muscle is usually a circular muscle that surrounds an opening, such as the pyloric sphincter that controls the emptying of the stomach, the sphincter vesicae or urethral sphincter that controls the emptying of the bladder and the anal sphincter. The urethral or bladder sphincter is a donut-shaped muscle just below the bladder neck. The base of the prostate is intimately connected to the primary sphincter. It may be difficult to determine where the sphincter ends and the prostate begins. So it is often damaged during a removal of the prostate.

Men have two sphincters that control the urine. The main or primary valve is the sphincter vesicae just below the bladder. It is also sometimes called the internal sphincter. The second valve is a musculo-membraneous sphincter just below the prostate. This sphincter is sometimes called the external valve or sphincter. Nature did not necessarily design it to control urine flow. If it was not damaged during the radical prostatectomy, it can be trained to work fairly well to control the urine after a prostatectomy.

KEGEL EXERCISES

Since women don't have a prostate, they have a very short urethra. They have a very rudimentary musculomembraneous sphincter which blends in with their primary bladder sphincter. They have far more incontinence problems than men. If you don't believe this, just go into any drugstore and check the many shelves that are stocked with adult diapers such as Depends and Attends. Most of these products are purchased by women.

Kegel exercises can strengthen the musculomembraneous sphincter and the pubococcygeus muscles of the pelvic floor. This can help shut off and control the urine flow.

Dr. Arnold H. Kegel, a gynecologist, developed the exercises for his women patients who were having incontinence problems. He would have the women start and stop the flow of urine while seated on the toilet with their legs spread wide apart. Once they had learned which muscles to control, he would ask them to exercise these muscles up to 300 times during each day. This strengthened the pubococcygeus muscle so that many of them overcame their incontinence.

Many of the women were surprised to find that the exercises greatly improved their sexual pleasure and contributed to their attainment of orgasm. The women's sexual partners also received the benefits of added pleasure due to women's exercise. They were able to squeeze and tighten the vaginal muscles at will.

Here is a quote from the *Encyclopedia and Dictionary of Medicine, Nursing and Allied Health, 2nd Edition*, published by W.B. Saunders Co.:

> "Research has since demonstrated that this muscle (the pubococcygeus) has specialized nerve endings which contribute to a satisfactory sexual experience...Once the muscle has been strengthened it tends to maintain its strength and state of partial contraction at all times. Sexual activity helps to preserve the muscle tone."

Men who have incontinence problems can also benefit from the Kegel exercises. To learn which muscles to strengthen, practice stopping the flow of urine several times. Then during the day clamp and hold the muscles tight for five to ten seconds. The exercises should be done at least 100 times per day. It would be even better to do 300 per day. These muscle exercises can allow the men to have a considerable amount of control over the movement of the penis, especially when it is erect. This muscle control can add to the pleasure of both male and female during the sex act.

The exercises can be done while watching TV, driving a car, sitting in church, or anywhere at any time. No one but you will know that you are doing them.

We spoke earlier about the fact that the primary bladder valve closed tightly when a man has an erection. This is so that the semen would be forced out of the end of the penis instead of taking the shorter route into the bladder. We also noted that the secondary musculomembraneous sphincter or secondary valve opens up when a man has an erection so that the semen can pass. This secondary valve usually closes down after a normal voiding of urine. This is the valve that lets you squeeze out the last few drops.

If a man has had a radical prostatectomy and the primary valve was severely damaged, it is usually possible for the man to regain normal control by using the Kegels to strengthen the secondary valve. This secondary musculomembraneous valve can be trained to control the normal voiding functions. But, since this valve has always opened up when a man has an erection, no amount of Kegels will cause it to remain closed when he has an erection or is even just trying to have an erection.

This may cause some very embarrassing situations if a man is preparing to have sex and he starts leaking urine. There may even be times when the man will start leaking if he has an erotic fantasy. One solution to the leaking problem is to use a rubber constriction ring such as those provided with vacuum erection devices (VEDs). Many of the men who have incontinence due to a radical prostatectomy, also have erectile dysfunction (ED) or impotence. So many of them must use the VEDs or some other aid in order to have intercourse. If they use some other form of aid, such as injections or Viagra, they may still have the urine leakage.

ANOTHER TYPE OF INCONTINENCE

Another type of incontinence that is rarely mentioned is fecal incontinence. One reason is because it is so embarrassing. Several men who have had radiation or some types of surgery have been left with the inability to control their feces. Kegel exercises may help in this situation, but usually, the nerves that control the anal sphincter have been damaged. So Kegels may not help much. There are also garments and pads that can be used for this problem.

PRODUCTS

Several companies manufacture undergarments for incontinence. Many of the materials are similar to the material used in baby diapers such as Huggies and Pampers. These two companies developed products with plastic outer layer and a layer of material that turns into a gel when it gets wet. The material can hold a large amount of liquid without leaking.

When first developed, both companies sued each other for infringement of patents. The judge who heard the case examined the products from both companies and refused to make a decision. He said that both cases seemed to hold water.

The same companies who make the baby diapers, also make the adult diapers or pads such as Attends and Depends. We have a listing of companies and products at the end of this chapter.

HUMOR ON THE INTERNET

Sometimes we get a bit bored on the Internet and we resort to the lowest form of humor, namely puns.

Bob Southard wrote: Those radical prostatectomy guys are RP'ers. (Our pee-ers).

Aubrey Pilgrim wrote back: Shame on you Bob. Urine in a lot of trouble!

Then George Orick chimed in from France: Aubrey, Bob, aren't we all going off the deep ends here? (Depends).

DR. BARTON WACHS' ARTICLE ON INCONTINENCE

It has been estimated that up to 20 million Americans suffer from urinary incontinence. Many of these are men who have undergone treatment for their prostate cancer. Simply stated, urinary incontinence is the inability to control the storage, or, for that matter, the release of urine. Normally, the urinary sphincter muscle controls the outflow of urine. When the abdominal pressure or bladder pressure overcomes the urethral pressure, incontinence ensues.

In men, the urinary sphincter muscle is located just below the bladder, surrounding the urethra. During radical prostate surgery, the prostate is removed, and the urethra, as well as the sphincters, are often damaged. The fine nerves adjacent to the urethra and prostate can also be damaged and thereby cause some form of incontinence. These nerves may also be damaged during radiation or cryosurgery.

The incidence of incontinence after radical surgery or radiation may be increased if one has had any of several problems. Neurologic problems such as multiple sclerosis may increase the risk of incontinence. The risk would be increased if the patient has undergone a stroke in the past, had a spinal cord injury or had surgery on the spine. A prior TURP may lead to incontinence after brachytherapy.

Urinary incontinence after cancer surgery or radiation is a significant and often devastating problem for both patients as well as the physicians. In this chapter, I will try to limit my comments to the involuntary loss of urine, or incontinence, after radical prostatectomy. Post-prostatectomy incontinence (PPI) is more common than incontinence after radiation therapy. The condition of incontinence can be temporary, mild, moderate, or permanent.

If you have an element of urinary incontinence after your surgery, it does not necessarily mean that your surgeon had a problem or performed the surgery wrong. It simply means that either the nerves, the sphincter, bladder neck, or even the bladder may have been altered as a result of the procedure. Purely from a statistical standpoint, the younger the patient, the better the continence after surgery.

PHYSIOLOGY OF MALE INCONTINENCE

There are three components responsible for continence in men. Of course, the bladder is important since it stores the urine. There is an internal or primary urinary sphincter that consists of the circular bladder neck muscles. The urethra itself provides a passive continence mechanism. The pelvic floor muscles include the striated rhabdosphincter or musculomembraneous sphincter. This sphincter is also sometimes called the external sphincter. It is primarily responsible for continence after prostate surgery.

The bladder neck can be rebuilt after the prostate is severed from the urethra, but the passive urethral mechanism is therefore altered. After prostate surgery, the internal sphincter, or those circular muscles around the bladder neck, are rendered incompetent. Just about the entire continence mechanism depends on the remaining muscles in the pelvic floor, or the external sphincter, and the urethra itself.

Medications that are sometimes given after prostate surgery to improve continence act on the nerve fibers around the external sphincter.

CAUSES OF POST PROSTATECTOMY INCONTINENCE (PPI)

The most obvious cause of post prostatectomy incontinence is that of damage to the sphincter muscle, as mentioned above. There are less obvious causes such as bladder and bladder neck obstruction or fibrosis, or a decompensated bladder, which is essentially a bladder that does not squeeze urine out well. One may also have problems if there is bladder instability, where the muscle or detrusor around the bladder becomes spasmotic.

There may also be neurologic causes of incontinence such as dementia, post stroke and Parkinson disease, and most worrisome, malignant infiltration of the sphincter mechanism.

Be sure your urologist rules out urinary tract infection. Having a catheter for up to two or more weeks while the urethral anastomosis heals may cause many patients to have mild to moderate urinary tract infection. The catheter may also cause irritation of the bladder neck and urethra.

There are various medicines that can exacerbate, or make worse, minimal urinary incontinence. Any sort of irritant to the bladder itself, bladder nerves, or urethra can cause urinary incontinence, urinary frequency urge to void, and urge incontinence. When speaking of incontinence, one must always take into consideration any concomitant illness, including neurologic disorder, age of the patient, and surgical procedure.

Comparing radical prostatectomies done from the retropubic position or the perineal position, there were no statistical differences in incontinence rates.

Nerve-sparing techniques have allowed a much more careful anatomic dissection and therefore less blood loss during a radical prostatectomy. This allows better visualization when reconnecting the urethral stump to the bladder after removing the prostate.

Hardly a month goes by without an article in the Journal of Urology talking about yet another surgical technique to minimize urinary incontinence. There are new surgical devices, new catheters, and harmonic scalpels that can improve the surgical technique and therefore improve the continence rate.

CaverMap, (which was discussed in Chapter 9 on Radical Prostatectomy) is a device that will make nerve sparing a lot easier. It should also improve on the incontinence rates.

After radical prostatectomy, if the margins are positive for cancer, one may consider radiation therapy. In this scenario, the risk of incontinence after radical prostatectomy and receiving radiation is about 5% to 15%.

DIAGNOSIS AND EVALUATION OF PPI

The evaluation of post-prostatectomy incontinence (PPI) usually consists of cystoscopy and urodynamics. Cystoscopy is looking into the bladder through a lighted flexible tubular telescope. Urodynamics is essentially the placement of a catheter and a pressure transducer, then measuring certain parameters, as well as the leak-point pressure. Both these procedures need to be combined with a thorough history to be sure that other pathologic conditions be addressed such as neurologic causes unrelated to the surgery. Also medical causes, such as diabetes, lumbar disk disease, and generally the aging process should be taken into consideration.

Urethral strictures or bladder strictures after surgery and residual obstructive tissue can also cause or make worse the PPI.

KEGEL EXERCISE FOR INCONTINENCE

You may ask what can be done to minimize the incidence of incontinence after surgery. One of the most simple maneuvers is simply to become proficient at Kegel exercises. (Kegel exercises were discussed earlier in this chapter).

Kegel exercises were popularized in women to improve their continency rates. Men can also benefit from these exercises. Even before the actual surgery is performed, I teach men how to control their sphincter.

The best way to learn the Kegel exercises is to practice while urinating. That is to say, while you are standing up, start and stop your urinary stream during the midstream. Try to isolate and snug up the muscles and hold on to these for at least four or five seconds. No one really is going to know whether you are doing these exercises correctly, and therefore, biofeedback and pelvic stimulation machines sometimes provide the answer. It is reasonable to perform these exercises up to 15 times a day to strengthen these muscles if they have been traumatized by surgery.

Do not lose patience if you find yourself incontinent after your catheter comes out. Many men have at least partial incontinence up to a year after the surgery. Therefore it is important to continue to perform the Kegel exercises. I advise against any surgery, such as for an artificial sphincter, until all other alternatives have been tried.

ELECTRICAL KEGELS

You may be shocked to know that most muscles can be stimulated to contract with an electrical signal. Some men and women have trouble identifying the proper muscles for performing the Kegel exercises correctly. Several years ago an electronic vaginal probe was developed for women.

After insertion into the vagina, a small voltage is sent to the probe which causes the pelvic floor muscles to contract. The same pelvic floor muscles can be stimulated from the rectum. So this probe can also be used by men. The advantage of the electrical stimulation is that the proper muscles needed for Kegels are always caused to contract.

Several companies manufacture these devices. The Empi Urologic Companyis one of the foremost and largest.

Here is some information about the Empi products from their web site: Empi, Inc. develops, manufactures and markets noninvasive biomedical devices and accessories for use in the orthopedic rehabilitation and incontinence treatment markets.

Minnova and Innova are easy-to-use battery operated stimulation devices designed for use with a vaginal or rectal electrode.   Recommended treatment is done in the privacy of the home for 15 minutes twice a day, every other day.   Clinical studies using pelvic floor stimulation have demonstrated cure and improvement rates of up to 73%.

CAUTION: Federal law (USA) restricts this device to sale by or on order of a physician.

To find out more, visit their web site at http://www.empi.com/

The Hollister Company also has a Pelvic Floor stimulator and other incontinence products. Hollister has been serving health care professionals and patients for more than 77 years. U.S.: 1.800.323.4060 Canada: 1.800.263.7400. http://www.hollister.com/

OTHER TREATMENTS FOR INCONTINENCE

The following are some other treatments for incontinence:

1. Absorption pads.
2. Biofeedback and Pelvic Stimulation
3. Medications.

4. Condom catheter.

5. Penile clamps.

6. Collagen, Teflon (Duraphase) and fat injections.

7. Artificial Urinary Sphincter.

MALE UNDERGARMENTS

Male undergarments are an effective way to absorb the urine that leaks. There are new types of undergarments that can effectively absorb this urine and decrease the smell. Undergarments together with medications and biofeedback may provide an effective way to control urinary incontinence. (Some of the companies are listed at the end of this chapter.)

BIOFEEDBACK

Biofeedback is an effective way of controlling incontinence. It is particularly effective when the incontinence is minimal and there is an urgency component secondary to either bladder instability, detrusor instability, or pelvic floor muscle abnormalities.

Biofeedback can be done passively, actively, and together with pelvic stimulation. Many urologists and physical therapists now have biofeedback machines. In my office I have a biofeedback machine and pelvic floor stimulator that is rather easy to use for the doctor, nurse, and the patient. It actually shows the patient that he is controlling the proper muscles and isolating the pelvic muscles instead of the entire abdominal wall muscles.

MEDICATIONS

There are several medications that can be tried, but only a few that seem to be effective. These medications are the ones that act on the bladder neck and the pelvic floor muscles.

Medications such as decongestants are most effective. Sudafed, Entex, or Ornade seem to help by controlling or snugging up the urethral and pelvic floor muscles. If the incontinence is minimal, these medicines may be effective. If there is an urge component or some bladder instability, other medications seem to be effective, such as Ditropan, Pro-Banthine, Levsin and Detrol. These medicines act to relax the bladder, while the decongestants strengthen or tighten the sphincter muscles.

Be careful of certain medications in that they can alter and elevate your blood pressure. When trying medications, remember that the therapeutic dose and the toxic dose may be closely associated. Please do not make your problem worse than the treatment.

CONDOM CATHETER

There are a few other treatment modalities, such as the use of a condom catheter, that can be tried. As the name implies, the condom catheter is a condom that fits over the penis. They are usually held in place with some type of adhesive. There are several different types and sizes. For slight leakage, there are some that have an extension for collection of the urine. For more serious leakage, the condom may have a nipple so that a hose and leg bag can be attached.

PENILE CLAMPS

Penile clamps have been around for a hundred years. They are still an effective way of controlling leakage. They are not my first choice because they are somewhat obtrusive and can cause problems if you leave them on too long. Some men who depend on these clamps forget to do their Kegel exercises, and this lack of motivation can, in fact, be a hindrance to learning to recontrol your muscles. In my practice, I discourage men from using these penile clamps unless all else fails.

COLLAGEN TREATMENTS

The use of collagen, a protein extract of connective tissue, can be injected adjacent to the urethra by a syringe under cystoscopic guidance. This is an extremely safe and easy treatment that can be performed under a local anesthesia. The problem is that collagen only works in selective cases. Collagen is much more effective in treating women with urinary stress incontinence than it is in men who have had prostatectomies.

Your own fat can also be used instead of collagen. The fat can be harvested through a technique that is similar to liposuction and then reinjected into the urethral tissues just like the collagen would be. Fat, of course, is much cheaper but probably not any more effective. After three to four collagen or fat injections, one should begin seeing control of the incontinence. It is my belief that after four collagen or fat injections and no results, this type of therapy should be abandoned. It is also important to note that collagen and fat injections are usually transient—the body absorbs them—so they only work for a period of months.

THE ARTIFICIAL URINARY SPHINCTER (AUS)

When all else fails, one can try to correct the incontinence by surgery. In my opinion, the artificial urinary sphincter is the gold standard by which all other treatments should be judged.

The artificial urinary sphincter is a device made from silicone. The silicone reservoir, however, is filled with sterile water or saline, and therefore there is no danger with regards to the silicone such as has been reported with breast implants.

The sphincter is made up of a reservoir, or bulb, that is implanted underneath the stomach muscles, a pump that is placed in the scrotum adjacent to the testicle, and the cuff which is placed around the urethra. There have been over 15,000 artificial urinary sphincters placed since 1984. Medical studies report an average continence success of over 90% in properly selected patients. With the use of kink-resistant tubing, postoperative problems have been brought down to a minimum. The malfunction rate of urinary sphincters has also significantly dropped since the kink-resistant tubing and deactivation have been instituted. The cuffs are low pressure and do not generally cause a problem with erosion or significant pressure problems, although this can be a factor.

The surgery takes less than an hour, and in my practice, is performed on an outpatient basis. Of course, the sphincter is not visible outside the body; so no one would know whether you have one or not.

The sphincter is released or deactivated by squeezing the pump. Urine then flows from the bladder, out the urethra normally. Within a few minutes, the cuff around the urethra, or the sphincter, automatically closes, keeping the urine from spilling from the bladder.

In a recent article in 1996 in the Journal of Urology, it was concluded that the artificial urinary sphincter was an effective form of therapy for post-radical-prostatectomy incontinence.

Patients were generally quite pleased with the sphincter, and the study revealed that 90% of these patients were satisfied and had marked improvement in their control.

The urinary sphincter is made by the American Medical Systems (AMS) a division of Pfizer Company. (AMS is the same company who makes the penile prosthesis.) It is a surgically implantable prosthesis used to restore bladder control. It is usually recommended for people who, because of injury, do not have a working sphincter or for people who have had other forms of treatment or surgery which have not been successful.

The artificial sphincter is implanted by your urologist inside the body but outside of the bladder. The cuff is placed around the urethra, in between the bladder and where the prostate was removed. The pump is placed in the scrotal sac. It is located just under the surface of the skin; so it is easily grasped. The reservoir or balloon is placed in the abdomen, under the muscles.

HOW DOES IT WORK?

The cuff is essentially a collar that squeezes the urethra shut to keep urine in the bladder. In order to pass urine from the bladder, the pump is squeezed in the scrotal sac, thereby releasing the cuff, and then the urine is passed from the bladder through the urethra. After a few minutes the cuff automatically reinflates and pressure is again placed around the urethra.

To help you understand how this device keeps you dry, imagine the cuff around the urethra is like a string around the neck of a balloon. When the string is tight around the neck of the balloon, no air can escape.

For more information about the artificial urinary sphincter, you can write to the American Medical Systems at 11001 Bren Road East, Minnetonka, Minnesota 55343, or call 1-800-328-3881. http://www.visitams.com/products/index.asp

SATISFACTION SURVEY

Here is a post on the internet from Russ Ingram, a young man who was diagnosed with prostate cancer at 39. He had a radical prostatectomy and hormone treatments. He was totally incontinent until he had an AUS:

Date: Mon, 3 Feb 1997

From: Russ D. Ingram

Subject: AUS Survey

I received a newsletter today from The National Association For Continence. (Their web site http://www.nafc.org). The part that was of interest to me in the newsletter is a report on a long term study of the QOL with the artificial urinary sphincter. Reports were for 68 men with an average follow-up of 7 years. Here are the results, based on a 0 to 5 scale with 5 being best: Degree of improvement 4.1, Degree of satisfaction 3.9.

Mine was implanted in May 96. I would give it a rating of 6 on a 0 to 5 scale. I was almost completely incontinent before. My QOL is so much better after AUS implant.

Till later

Russell

RUSS INGRAM LOST THE BATTLE

Russ put up a valiant fight, but lost the battle. He died on Dec. 28, 1998. He was 46 years old. He left a loving wife, two daughters, and a son.

BE INFORMED

Taking all things into consideration, one should not go into radical prostate surgery without knowing about the incidence of incontinence and impotence. However, controlling the spread of cancer or removing the prostate cancer should be of foremost importance when deciding on a type of therapy.

In the future, there will be new forms of therapy to control urinary incontinence after prostatectomy. In Europe the use of poly-Teflon has proved effective as a bulking agent when used instead of collagen.

Silicone has also been used. Unlike the collagen and fat, these agents are not absorbed and removed by the body so they last for sometime. However, the FDA has not approved the use of these substances in the U.S. Maybe they will be approved in the future.

RESOURCES FOR INCONTINENCE PRODUCTS

There are several organizations and companies who specialize in providing information and products for incontinent patients.

The National Association For Continence

Mission: National Association For Continence (NAFC) was formerly known as Help for Incontinent People (HIP). The NAFC is a not-for-profit organization dedicated to improving the quality of life of people with incontinence. NAFC's purpose is to be the leading source of education, advocacy and support to the public and to the health professional about the causes, prevention, diagnosis, treatments, and management alternatives for incontinence. Funding: NAFC's activities are funded primarily by voluntary contributions from consumers, health professionals, and industry.

NAFC's challenges are to destigmatize incontinence, to provide consumer information, and to provide advocacy and service for those who are affected by this problem. NAFC offers:

Quality Care a quarterly newsletter that provides moral support and practical information to over 100,000 subscribers.

The *Resource Guide*—Products and Services for Incontinence, which assists people in finding the most helpful product for their type of incontinence.

Pamphlets, audio/visuals, and books designed to educate the general public and health care professionals.

Established: 1982, Founder: Katherine F. Jeter, EdD
Mailing Address: P.O. Box 8310, Spartanburg, SC 29305-8306
Telephone: 864-579-5700; Fax: 864-579-7902
Toll-Free HelpLine: 1-800-BLADDER (800-252-3337)

OTHER RESOURCES

The Simon Foundation For Continence

P.O Box 835, WILMETTE, ILL 60091.

Free information packet; Books, videos, tapes, quarterly news-letters (with $15 membership fee) support group referrals. Phone 800 23-SIMON.

TransAqua

The TransAqua system has a Health Dri system of washable bladder control garments. They have several different types that are suitable for moderate to severe incontinence.

Phone 1-800-769-1899 for brochures and more information.
www.trans-aqua.com

Allstate Medical Products

Allstate has a large selection of undergarments, pads and linens. They are washable so they are long lasting. See fig. 17-3

1-800-322-1123 for a product catalog.

INTERNET SITES FOR INCONTINENCE

I did a search of the Internet for incontinence and got almost 100 different sites. Here are a few that offer products and information. To access one of the sites, log on to your Internet, then simply highlight the URL, then use Control + C to copy, place your cursor in the browser area of your online Internet and press Control + V to place URL text in the Browser area.

http://www.everythingmedical.com/

There are many web sites for incontinence supplies and products. Use the Internet search engines such as www.google.com, www.yahoo.com, www.excite.com, www.lycos.com, www.altavista.com and any of the others.

We wish you all the best and that you stay dry.

Chapter Sixteen

ERECTILE DYSFUNCTION

By Drs. Stephen Auerbach and Aubrey Pilgrim

Stephen M. Auerbach, MD is a urologist who specializes in the treatment of impotence and male erectile dysfunction. He has worked in private practice in Newport Beach, California since 1980. Dr. Auerbach has been involved in clinical research of all of the medications which have recently gained FDA approval for the treatment of impotence. He currently is conducting clinical studies on the new medications discussed in this chapter.

Dr. Auerbach is a founding member of Affiliated Research Centers which is a nationwide clinical research group. He is the Medical Advisor for Impotents' Anonymous, a support group for impotent men and their partners. Dr. Auerbach has worked as a consultant for many pharmaceutical companies helping them develop their clinical research protocols. He has also trained urologists on new surgical techniques in the treatment of impotence. As you will see in this section of the book, he stresses the emotional impact of this medical problem. He always prefers to get the patient's wife or partner involved in the treatment plan in order to achieve the best results.

Dr. Auerbach has authored a previous impotence book, entitled, "*Partners In Overcoming Impotence.*" He has produced audio tapes entitled, "*Prostate Solutions*" and "*Lifelong Potency*" which have patient and partner interviews discussing the impact of these very personal problems.

DEDICATION

Impotence affects over 30 million men and their partners. This part of the book is dedicated to all those men and their partners who are either facing the fear of possible impotence associated with the treatment of prostate cancer, or those who are already experiencing erectile difficulties. Impotence is a problem which can be very devastating, not only to the man, but also to his partner. It is difficult enough facing the diagnosis and treatment of prostate cancer. However, having to worry about a possible impotence problem makes the whole situation more complex, difficult and overwhelming.

I hope that this information will provide encouragement to all those men who have been afraid to seek help. Even if you have already asked your doctor for help and have not gotten an answer, don't be discouraged.

A FATE WORSE THAN DEATH

Erectile dysfunction (ED) used to be called impotence, but the euphemism ED doesn't seem as harsh. A few years ago we had no treatments for ED. Even if he was the richest man in the world, if he couldn't get an erection, there was nothing that could be done. Sex, the drive to propagate the species, is the strongest drive in man or animal. It is your one path to immortality. Half of each offspring comes from you. So the more offspring, the more of you is left behind. Some considered impotence to be a fate worse than death.

I have no doubt that even some of the early cavemen had ED. Even kings and the lowest slaves sometimes suffered from it. All kinds of witches brews, potions and drugs were tried. Few, if any, worked. Today we have several ways to treat ED, including vacuum erection devices, drugs and prostheses for penile implants.

HELP IS AVAILABLE.

Today there are several solutions. The most important message is that impotence, the inability of a man to achieve and maintain an erection suitable for vaginal intercourse, is one of the few diseases that can almost always be successfully treated. These are very exciting times for the impotent man and his partner. In 1998, Viagra received FDA approval and changed the way we look and talk about erection problems. Viagra made it OK to discuss this devastating problem.

Numerous other medications are undergoing investigation and are on the drawing board. Impotence can be treated and fixed! There is hope.

IMPOTENCE IS THE UNSPOKEN TOPIC

Finding a doctor is a very difficult process for most men suffering from ED. Men generally do not talk about private issues. They especially do not like to talk about erectile problems. Many physicians are not aware of the different treatment alternatives and do not feel comfortable treating impotence. Also, many doctors don't look at ED as a real medical problem when they are taking care of men suffering from medical issues such as heart attack, hypertension, diabetes, etc.

ED is not a typical subject that a man discusses with another person. It is difficult for the patient and difficult for the doctor. Physicians frequently feel uncomfortable talking about this problem. Many doctors don't have the time or emotional energy to get involved in the treatment of ED.

A man may find it much easier to tell his work associates or a family member that he has been diagnosed with the prostate cancer or had a heart attack, than telling them about an erectile problem. ED is a taboo subject in our society. However, ED or impotence, affects every part of a man's life. Impotence is critical to a man's ego and self-image.

THE IMPORTANCE OF ERECTILE FUNCTION

Sex is extremely important in our society. Sex has gone from being the way of carrying on our species, by having children, to being the way we express ourselves as accepted men and women in our society today. We are one of the few species of animals that has sex for pure pleasure. Excluding the dolphins and man, every other specie has sexual relations only to reproduce offspring.

The act of sexual relations is not just a necessity to carry on the life blood of the species, it is a pleasurable encounter. It is a way of adding value to our lives and gives couples an added feeling of well-being, closeness, and acceptance.

DELAY IN SEEKING TREATMENT

Most men think their erectile difficulties will be a fleeting problem that will go away on their own. They are told that it may take up to a year for their erectile activity to return following radical prostate surgery or radiation. Frequently, the erectile function will improve, but in many cases ED due to nerve or vascular injury may be permanent. It is a mistake to wait. The earlier the treatment, the more likely the success.

NOCTURNAL ERECTIONS

The penis is a vascular organ that requires regular blood flow or "exercise." There is something to the statement, "Use it or lose it!." Normally men experience nocturnal or night-time erections while they are sleeping. They may experience 3 to 5 erections associated with REM (Rapid Eye Movement) sleep. These erections may last up to one hour or more in time. They are important for oxygenating or exercising the penile erectile tissue.

Research by Dr. Irwin Goldstein of Boston University has shown that men who experience these night-time erections have more smooth muscle in their penises, which is necessary to trap blood in the penis during the erection process. Men who do not achieve nighttime erections may have the smooth muscle in their penis replaced with collagen or scar tissue. The collagen is not able to trap the blood in the penis, and thus the man will experience erectile failure. This is especially common following injury to the nerves and blood vessels of the penis associated with the treatment of prostate cancer.

PSYCHOLOGICAL AND OTHER CAUSES OF IMPOTENCE

Our brain is the most important sexual organ that we have. And there are hundreds of ways for the brain to cause our sexual apparatus not to operate at an optimum performance. There are many things that can cause a psychogenic erectile dysfunction. The psychogenic ED may be only temporary or may be permanent. A man may suffer ED with one partner, but be okay with someone else. There may also be many problems such as finances, work, health problems and dozens of other things that may cause psychogenic ED.

There can be psychological impotence associated with having cancer of the prostate. Following the diagnosis and/or treatment, many men experience fear of the illness and their own mortality. They may be depressed and really not be able to perform sexually. Men suffering from depression are at four times greater incidence of impotence than men without depression. Men with hypertension and diabetes are at two times greater risk of developing ED.

Most men expect their bodies to respond like machines. They may be fearful to even pursue sexual contact following their treatment for the fear of failure, possible injury to the treated area, or even embarrassment of possible side effects, such as urinary incontinence. Because of these fears, some men may actually avoid sexual contact.

Even if the man still has some erectile function, the fear of possible failure may actually cause him to develop psychological impotence. The anxiety and stress would cause him to be unable to achieve and maintain an erection.

Fear causes our bodies to secrete adrenaline which may be necessary for our survival in case of emergency. Adrenaline causes increased blood flow to the vital organs necessary for survival.

There is increased blood flow to the heart, brain, and muscles. Our hearts pound faster and stronger, we become more alert, and our muscles get the necessary blood flow to deliver oxygen so that our body can respond to the danger and increased demand put on them.

At the same time, blood is shunted away from the nonvital organs such as our stomach, intestines, and penis. Though these organs are important, they are not vital for the immediate survival of our species. Therefore, we actually experience a physical response from a psychological event.

After experiencing an erectile failure, the man often expects failure the next time he tries to engage in sexual activity. The man may hope the problem will get better on its own. But by delaying treatment, a small problem may become much bigger and more difficult to treat. At some point in time, the man will expect to fail on every attempt at sexual intercourse. At this time the problem may become much more significant.

FEARFUL OF TREATMENT OPTIONS

Every man wishes that there was a magic potion, lotion or pill he could take which would reinvigorate his sexual appetite and ability. If this type of medication is ever discovered there will be an acute shortage immediately because even normal-functioning men would want to buy it to improve and insure their sexual functioning.

From early times, there has been tremendous concern by men about their sexual functioning. The search for the magic potion or cure has been a top priority. Ginseng tea has been touted as a sexually enhancing brew. The rhinoceros has almost been hunted to extinction since the 15th century because men thought its horn would make them horny. The Chinese thought the ground-up horn offered potent strengths and qualities to whoever took it. Unfortunately, none of these things help very much. The magic potion still eludes us.

With the release of Viagra, we have opened the door of maintaining sexual vitality throughout our lives. Viagra is not an aphrodisiac, but it is a medicine that helps to assist and maintain blood flow to the penile tissue. Unfortunately, it does not work in all men, especially those whose erectile nerves were removed or severely damaged due to a prostatectomy or other cancer treatments.

Prior to Viagra, when patients were told of the different treatment options, they usually were not pleased with the choices. One patient said, "When I was told that I needed a penile implant I felt that this was too drastic a step and I sought help elsewhere. I was happy to find out there were other options. I received a full work-up and found that medication could help me."

Other patients are not pleased with the thought of having to use a needle for penile injection therapy. But whatever the treatment, patients must realize that this is a solvable problem. They should investigate the options and get the advice of a qualified urologist who is knowledgeable about erectile problems and have a proper diagnostic work-up.

If at all possible, talk to patients who have undergone some of the available treatments. Today, with chat rooms and mailing lists on the Internet, this becomes possible. A good mailing list for sexual questions is at PCAI (which stands for Prostate Cancer And Intimacy). For a free subscription, send e-mail to:

> majordomo@prostatepointers.org
> Subject: leave blank
> Message: Subscribe PCAI

ACHIEVING SUCCESS

1. Gather information

Information helps you to regain your power. At one time the subject of impotence and erectile dysfunction (ED) was seldom mentioned. But information is available everywhere today. There are articles on the Internet about every form of therapy available. Use any search engine such as www.google.com, www.yahoo.com, www.excite.com, www.lycos.com, or any of the other search engines and search for erectile dysfunction. You will find dozens of sites. At the American Urological Association (AUA) meeting in 2000, there 89 abstracts presented regarding ED and/or Sexual Dysfunction. There were six papers presented on Female Sexual Dysfunction (FSD).

The subject of ED is now often discussed on radio and TV shows. Numerous articles and books are in print. There are a few Impotents' Anonymous support groups for patients and their partners.

The following resources can be helpful in finding a qualified doctor who is knowledgeable of the latest medical therapies for the treatment of impotence.

Here is an excellent Internet site: www.hisandherhealth.com/

Another very good site is Impotence FAQ: http://www.palace.net/~llama/asifaq.html

This site has a resources section for autoinjectors and lots of other information.

Another good site is this one: http://www.phoenix5.org. It was put together by Robert Young to help men and their companions with the deeply personal issues created by prostate cancer. He was diagnosed 11/23/99 with a PSA 1000+. The Impotence Institute of America & Impotence Anonymous at (800)-669-1603 is a very good resource. They publish a newsletter with all of the latest ED information.

I have an excellent tape, entitled, "*Lifelong Potency*", which discusses all of the causes of impotence, diagnostic treatment options and therapies. This can be purchased through my office at: 400 Newport Center Drive, Suite 501, Newport Beach, CA. 92660 Tel: 714-644-7200 Cost $14.95 + Shipping

2. Ask For Help

Finding a doctor can be very difficult for most men. It may be difficult for a man to gather the courage to ask for help. And frequently, when he does ask his doctor for help, he is met with less than a satisfying answer. Many doctors are not knowledgeable of the different treatments that are available. Moreover, many of them do not consider ED a real medical problem.

I lead an Impotents Anonymous meeting which discusses any issue surrounding male sexual dysfunction and impotence. We get 40-60 men and their partners to each meeting. Many of them feel very nervous, uncomfortable and anxious when they first come to these meetings. A real good icebreaker for us is to ask the question, "Has anyone ever asked their doctor for help?" Usually 45-50 men will raise their hands. When I ask them, "Did you get an adequate answer to your problem?" Only one or two men leave their hands in the air.

Following this question, everyone realizes that they are on common ground. It is very painful for a man to ask for help regarding this very private subject. He is embarrassed and shamed. When he is left hanging with a less than helpful response, he may become even more discouraged.

The doctor should offer you all of the different treatment options discussed in this book. If a doctor only offers you surgery for penile implants or nothing, you have the wrong man or woman. Most men can be effectively treated medically. Surgical treatment should be the last option and not the first one.

3. Partner Involvement

It is important to have your partner involved in the treatment process. The more she understands about the causes and available treatment, the better the couple can work as a team. There will also be much better acceptance of the entire treatment process. However, in my experience, many men avoid getting their partners involved in the diagnostic and treatment process. They may feel vulnerable and ashamed.

Some men try to hide their ED from their wives. Frequently, men will avoid any physical contact that could lead to sexual activity. They go to bed earlier or later than their wives just to avoid contact. Perhaps the problem has already been present for sometime prior to the onset of prostate cancer. The whole process is very embarrassing to a man.

4. FOCUS ON THE PROBLEM AND SOLUTIONS

Be specific about your concerns. Write down any questions you may have. Concentrate on those issues that you can control. Don't waste your time and energy on extraneous topics. Your goal is to solve the problem of impotence. Do whatever it takes to be successful in this endeavor. Get all the information you can about the problem of impotence and more importantly, learn about the solutions.

I have found that many of the men I have treated focused much of their energies on the facts, costs, and potential problems. Very few men have really evaluated how their problem has hurt them or their relationship. It is so much easier for a man to look at the cold facts than to think about feelings. For this very reason, support groups such as Impotents Anonymous have been very successful. Call Impotence Institute of America & Impotence Anonymous at (800)-669-1603 and ask if there is a support group in your area.

These groups offer a forum where men and their partners can hear how the problem of ED affected others before and after treatment. Most men discover that there is hope through these meetings. Hearing how couples have successfully dealt with their impotence problem is extremely helpful for facing either the prospect of becoming impotent or those already experiencing the problem.

5. Choosing the most effective treatment

Keep an open mind about treatments—knowledge is power. Become informed. Learn about your options. There are many choices you can make. I tell my patients about the different options available to them after a diagnosis has been made. We usually start with the least invasive treatment option and progress to others if the less aggressive therapy fails.

Some men are fearful of the treatments, and the thought of regaining their sexual function alone is not enough to motivate them to treat their problem. Frequently, the potential loss of their self-esteem or a relationship will be the motivating factor that drives them into the doctor's office for help.

HITTING BOTTOM

Sometimes, so much water can pass under the bridge that there can be irreparable damage to a relationship. Communication between the partners can come to a standstill. There can be much arguing and fighting. Much anger and resentment can be expressed toward each other. Both men and women may have affairs to see if things will be better with someone else.

Often, one partner may blame the other for the cause of the problem. The final result can be separation and even divorce. Hopefully, the man and his partner will be directed to proper help so they don't have to hit bottom.

A recent study of 75 patients with organic impotence was performed by researchers Kristine Zurowski, Herbert Kayne, and Irwin Goldstein, M.D. Patients were asked questions about how impotence affected their life and behavior. The findings showed the following interesting results:

o Approximately 65% reported a decline in their self-esteem and self-confidence. (Personally, I think the number is closer to 90% or even 95% in the patients I have examined and treated).

o 71% reported increased levels of frustration.

o 61% reported increased anxiety.

o There were significant increases in smoking and drinking.

o One in four speculated that their impotence was a definite or possible factor in a break-up of a relationship.

A man will seek treatment when he has experienced enough pain and realizes and feels the impact of his problem. Action occurs when his pain and potential loss of his partner or self-esteem becomes greater than his fear and embarrassment associated with this problem and expected treatment.

IMPOTENTS' ANONYMOUS SUPPORT GROUP

Patients feel much better after attending an IA (Impotents' Anonymous) meeting. One patient stated, "Just that I had done something made me feel better. The fact that other people had worked through and were experiencing the same type of problems that I was going through made me feel better. I was not a freak. I was not alone."

The advantage for a patient attending an impotence support group is that both the man and his partner have the opportunity to learn about impotence. They not only learn factual information regarding impotence, but more importantly see and feel the effects of impotence on their lives.

The despair, sadness, pain, and most importantly the hope that there is life after an erectile problem can be solved. The experiences of others can be a facilitative tool to helping him seek help.

Women, on the other hand are more interested in the whole relationship and hearing about how other couples have solved their problems. Most women are concerned about the change in their partner's confidence and loss of closeness in their relationship. Some IA groups have separate IA-ANON groups where the women can meet to discuss their issues. There is a lot of support from patients who have already undergone treatment and this can be extremely helpful for the couple seeking an answer to their problem.

Again, call Impotence Institute of America & Impotence Anonymous at (800)-669-1603 and ask if there are any support groups in your area. If not, maybe you could start one. If you belong to a prostate cancer support group, you may be able to have several of the men and wives join an IA support group.

PHYSIOLOGY OF ERECTION

An erection is a vascular event. Our arteries are made up of tubular muscles in a closed system. By constricting the arteries in one area of the body, and relaxing them in another area, blood can be shifted to where it is most needed at that time. In the flaccid state, the arteries of the penis are in a constricted mode.

When a man thinks about sex, or is physically stimulated, nerve impulses are sent through the spinal cord to the penile tissue. This action results in the release of nitric oxide (NO). The NO causes a chemical reaction to form cyclic Guanosine Monophosphate (cGMP). The cGMP and NO causes a marked relaxation of the smooth arterial muscle and erectile tissues. The relaxation of the smooth muscle in the penile arteries allows an influx of arterial blood. The blood flows in faster than the veins can move it out. The expanding blood-filled spongy tissue compresses the veins against the sheath around the penis. This compression of the veins helps trap the blood in the penis and rigidity is achieved.

The body has a natural way to reverse this process. There is an enzyme called, Phosphodiesterase type 5, (PDE 5) which breaks down cGMP. Without the cGMP, there is no nitric oxide and the arteries again become constricted, the inflow of blood is reduced and the penis returns to its flaccid state. Viagra inhibits the PDE 5 and prevents the breakdown of cGMP.

THE ERECTILE NERVES

There is a bundle of nerves and blood vessels that lie along each side of the prostate. Quite often these nerves are severed or severely damaged during a radical prostatectomy when the prostate is removed. These are the nerves which cause the nitric oxide to be produced. Without these nerves, there will be no nitric oxide and cGMP and Viagra may have little or no effect. But even without the erectile nerves, some men have been able to have a partial effect from Viagra. Some men then use a vacuum erection device (VED) to create a firm erection.

DIAGNOSIS OF IMPOTENCE

History

The patient's history of his erectile problem is very significant and can help the physician make a proper diagnosis. First the doctor will want to know if the man is able to get any kind of erection with foreplay, masturbation, or upon awakening in the middle of the night or in the morning. Frequently, these night erections are noticed when the man has to get up to urinate in the middle of the night. These erections are associated with the dream phase of a man's sleep. This dream phase is called REM sleep. REM stands for "rapid eye movement." It is a positive sign if the man is capable of achieving any kind of erection at all.

If the man's impotence is secondary to the treatment of prostate cancer, he may give a history of having good erections prior to either surgery or radiation, and then noticed the onset of ED immediately after the treatment phase. Sometimes, if the erectile nerves were only damaged and not severed, he may slowly regain some or all of his function as time passes. Some men will see improvement up to one year following surgery.

Medications

Many medications can affect a man's erectile function. Most medications used for the treatment of hypertension and depression may inhibit the normal erectile response. Most of these medications inhibit normal erectile function by either decreasing the amount of blood reaching the penile chambers or working centrally in the brain by inhibiting the initiation of the erectile process. At times, the offending medication can be changed to an alternative medication that may result in a return to normal sexual function.

Hormone Therapy

Prostate cancer thrives on the male hormone, testosterone. Often the patient will be treated by combined hormonal blockade or an orchiectomy (surgical removal of the testicles). Without testosterone, there is loss of sexual libido. However, men may still be sexually active, using Viagra, MUSE, penile injections, the vacuum device or other treatments.

VIAGRA (SILDENAFIL) & COMPLETE ANDROGEN BLOCKADE

Drs. Scholz and Strum did a study of a few men who were on complete androgen blockade (CAB) and the use of Viagra. Most men who are on CAB have no libido, but they still have intact erectile nerves and blood supply so they should be able to attain erections.

The *Journal of Urology* printed their report in the June 1999 issue, page 1914. Drs. Scholz and Strum say, "It was the first...(study) to our knowledge on the efficacy of Viagra in patients with erectile dysfunction due to complete androgen blockade. We agree that in these patients the administration of sildenafil once or twice a week to facilitate sexual intercourse might be of importance in reducing the risk of prolonged cavernous tissue hypoxia and subsequent irreversible tissue damage." Again and again, use it or lose it. They only had 21 patients in the study, but it seemed to prove that men could have sex even with a castrate level of testosterone and no libido.

Reasons offered for wanting to use sildenafil varied and included regard for partner needs, enjoyment of intimacy and closeness, partner insistence and the concern, "use it or lose it." Regarding this latter motive, we have noted that physicians commonly fail to consider how protracted loss of nocturnal erections leads to irreversible erectile dysfunction. This problem needs to be addressed openly because intermittent combined androgen blockade is being used with increasing frequency for early stage prostate cancer.

Sildenafil induces erections of adequate quality for intercourse in men with castrate testosterone levels and may avert the development of penile atrophy if used regularly. We believe that the option of weekly or biweekly sildenafil should be discussed with patients on combined androgen blockade therapy as a possible means of averting future erectile dysfunction. Additionally, patients seem to benefit and be comforted by resumption of physical closeness during a difficult period of illness and uncertainty.

Mark Scholz and Stephen Strum Prostate Cancer Research Institute4676 Admiralty Way#101Marina del Rey, California 90292.

Editorial Note: If you are on CAB, the penile tissues will atrophy and shrink if the tissues do not receive nourishing blood occasionally. One of the better ways to do it is to use a vacuum erection device (VED). Even if you don't plan to use the erection for fun, you should use the device once in a while to keep the penis nourished.

MEDICAL RESEARCH OFFERS HOPE

For many years men have dreamed of a magic pill that would solve their impotence problems. With the release of Viagra, we have experienced valuable hope and help to the millions of men suffering from ED. Viagra is a medication which was originally designed to increase blood flow to the heart for men with angina or chest pain. During initial clinical trials, many men experienced unexpected erections. Viagra has been investigated in numerous clinical trials. Several million prescriptions have been written world-wide. A few men have died of heart attacks while on Viagra, but out of the millions who have used it, the number who died may have died if they were not using Viagra. Viagra has been shown to be efficacious and safe in the treatment of ED.

The clinical results have been successful in most men. Viagra has been shown to be effective in about 70% of men with organic impotence and up to 92% of men with psychogenic impotence. The most common side effects associated with the use of Viagra are:

Headache	16%
Flushing	10%
Indigestion	8%
Nasal Congestion	4%
Urinary Tract Infection	3%
Visual Disturbances	3%
Muscle Aches	1%

Most men also experience seeing a blue haze, almost like looking through blue colored glasses. It does not seem to cause any physical damage.

Patients receiving nitrates such as nitroglycerin in any form can NOT use Viagra under any circumstances. Combining Viagra with nitrates can result in a serious lowering of the blood pressure of up to 50 mmHg. This large drop in blood pressure can result in heart attack and death. Viagra is safe for men taking high blood pressure medications, Coumadin, anti-arrhythmic heart medications, and alcohol.

Studies show that Viagra does *not* increase the risk of serious cardiovascular event including heart attack over placebo. Exercise and stress on the heart is usually the cause of heart attack in men, not the Viagra.

Viagra should be taken with an empty stomach about 1 hour before planned sexual relations. To create an erection requires sexual stimulation. If a man is eating or drinking alcohol, he should wait 2 hours before engaging in sexual activity. Men should be relaxed when first using Viagra. A man must have physical or emotional readiness when using Viagra. We start patients on 50 mg of Viagra for 5 doses to see if it will work.They are increased to 100 mg if the results are not satisfactory.

Note that most pharmacies charge about the same for 100 mg as for the 50 mg. If you respond to 50 mg, you may be able to save money if you buy the 100 mg tablets, then use a pill splitter to cut them in half. Most pharmacies will sell you a pill splitter for a nominal amount.

VASOMAX (REGITINE OR PHENTOLAMINE)

Vasomax is another medication that works to increase penile blood flow. It is currently undergoing investigational clinical trials in the United States and world wide. The medication has previously been used for years to help with erections as an injectable medication. Recently, the manufacturer, Zonagen, Inc., in Texas, has developed an oral delivery system for this medication which is designed to work within about 10 minutes. It will be most useful in those men with mild vascular problems causing their erectile failure. It will probably not be effective in those men with severe erectile failure.

Vasomax is being developed by ScheringPlough and studies are waiting to resume.

The results at this time have not been very encouraging for this drug.

UPRIMA (APO-MORPHINE)

This is a medication manufactured by TAP Pharmaceuticals and is awaiting approval by the FDA. It was expected to be approved in late 2000, but it was delayed so that more tests could be done.

Apo-Morphine is being evaluated for the treatment of psychogenic and also organic impotence. It appears to work by blocking the adrenaline response initiated by the brain. Men with psychogenic impotence have the ability to achieve an erection but tend to lose it soon after starting intercourse because they are afraid of possibly failing. When a man has failed previously with sexual relations, his body will emit small doses of adrenaline and negative messages from his brain. From an emotional event, a physical response occurs. The adrenaline causes constriction of the penile arteries and subsequently there is loss of the erection.

Uprima (Apo-Morphine) blocks this adrenaline response pattern and has been shown to be most effective in some patients with psychogenic symptoms. The medication is taken sublingually (under the tongue) just prior to sexual relations. Uprima works within 15 minutes.

It is necessary to proceed with foreplay and then start the desired sexual activity. Uprima has been effective in certain groups of patients. The benefit of this medication is that it works quickly. The primary side effect has been nausea which has been seen in a small percentage of men. It was more common with higher doses, but further research shows that cutting back on the dose has worked well with fewer side effects.

OTHER NEW MEDICATIONS

Cialis from Lilly-ICOS

Lilly-ICOS has developed Cialis, a longer-acting medication similar to Viagra. This drug is also a Phosphodiesterase 5 (PDE-5) inhibitor. The Cialis medication has a longer half-life than Viagra and will work up to 24 hours after administration. This medication is expected to be approved by the FDA soon.

Many females also have sexual dysfunction. Females have been added to the ICOS clinical trials. Trials using Viagra on women are also ongoing.

Vardenafil from Bayer

Bayer is also working on Verdanafil, a Viagra-type medication. Verdanafil may last as long as 18 hours. Pfizer itself is also working on a newer, better PDE 5 inhibitor. Verdanafil is expected to be shortly approved by the FDA .

VACUUM ERECTION DEVICES

These are devices that work to create an erection mechanically. They consist of a hollow, cylindrical tube which is placed over the penis. There is a pumping device which creates a vacuum, thus drawing blood into the penis. Once the penis is enlarged and firm, an elastic ring device is released from the cylinder and is slipped onto the penis. The blood is then trapped in the penis, giving it rigidity. See Fig. 16-1.

The process was invented in the 1970s by Geddings Osbon Sr., a retired tire dealer and Pentecostal preacher who fashioned prototype devices from tire pumps.

When Geddings began marketing his ErecAid, the Post Office and several other government officials decided that the device and its instructional literature were pornographic and obscene. His devices that were sent through the mails were seized and he was threatened with fines and prison. The business was almost ended before it could get started.

Mr. Osbon was finally able to convince a few doctors of the benefits of the ErecAid and they began to prescribe it for their patients. There are now millions of patients who use vacuum devices. These devices allowed the impotent patients to finally enjoy the pleasures of sex. Several other companies besides Osbon are now selling devices that are essentially the same as the original Osbon device.

At one time you needed a prescription from your doctor to purchase one of these devices but several companies now offer them without a prescription. You will still need a prescription if you want your insurance company to pay for one. If you are a Medicare recipient, the government will even pay for it if you have a doctor's prescription.

The vacuum devices may cost from $79 from some companies and up to over $300. Some deluxe VEDs have a small motor to create the vacuum. These deluxe units may cost as much as $400 or more. Walmart and several drugstores now carry non-prescription units that cost about $120. You may also call 1-800-475-3091 or 888-231-2486 for units that cost about $80.

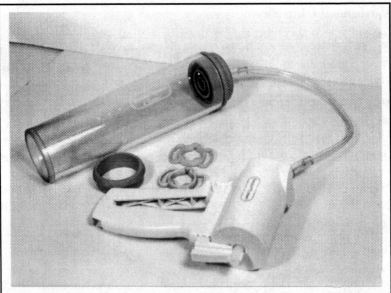

FIG. 16-1 An Osbon Vacuum Erection Device (VED)

The Osbon Company has a booklet called A Patient's Guide for the Treatment of Impotence. Call Osbon at 1-800-438-8592 for a copy of this informative booklet and a brochure about their ErecAid. They also have a web site at http://www.timmmedical.com/. The web site has photos and a vast amount of information about the VED.

Some of the rings are narrow and can be rather uncomfortable. Some companies, such as Mission Pharmacal at 800-531-3333, have developed rings that have a wide band that spreads the constriction over a wider area so that they are more comfortable. They have a web site with lots of information at http://www.missionpharmacal.com/.

There is an old expression, use it or lose it. If a man goes without an erection for a long time, the tissues in the penis may atrophy and the penis will shrink. Most men complain that they don't have enough already and don't want to lose any. The VED can bring fresh blood into the penis. Some men have even claimed to have enlarged their penis by regular daily use of the VED.

Many men have found these devices to be successful. The advantage is that there are no medications or invasive procedures. The disadvantage is that there is some preparation time and less spontaneity of the sexual act.

FDA APPROVES FIRST FEMALE SEXUAL AID DEVICE, EROS

The Food and Drug Administration (FDA) has approved the first prescription device designed to help women with sexual dysfunction problems.

The device, called the Eros Clitoral Therapy Device (CTD) works on the same principle as the vacuum pumps sold to help men achieve erections. It helps pump blood into the genital area.

It is made by Urometrics, a small, privately owned company in St. Paul, Minnesota. Female sexual arousal disorder (FSAD) is classified as a legitimate disease by the National Institute of Health and is characterized by one or more of the following symptoms: inability to experience an orgasm, lack of lubrication (often causing painful intercourse and/or lack of desire or decreased libido), and lack of clitoral sensation.

FSAD is often characterized by a lack of vaginal lubrication, painful intercourse and/or a reduced ability to achieve an orgasm. Certain physical conditions which cause constriction of the vaginal and clitoral arteries may interfere with or prevent a woman from achieving clitoral tumescence. It is believed that the difficulty or inability to achieve clitoral tumescence may be related to other symptoms of female sexual dysfunction such as: lack of desire, difficulty achieving orgasm, insufficient vaginal lubrication and painful intercourse.

Application of a vacuum over the female clitoris will cause clitoral engorgement and blood flow. FSAD and orgasmic disorder are believed to be related to reduced blood flow in the female genitalia.

It has been estimated that as many as 50 percent of U.S. women complain they have problems enjoying sex after they go through menopause. These problems can be physically measured and often have to do with decreased blood flow to the genital area—the same physical problem that underlies many cases of erectile dysfunction.

To find out more about the Eros-CTD go to: www.urometrics.com

About one third of the penis is within the man's body and most of the clitoris is also within the female's body. The actual length of the entire clitoris may be almost four inches long.

There is an informational site designed for women and their partners who have questions and concerns about women's sexual health at:

http://www.womenssexualhealth.com/

MUSE (MEDICAL URETHRAL SYSTEM FOR ERECTION)

This is a product developed by Vivus Corporation in California. It is a small cream pellet with the active component being Prostaglandin E1. The pellet dissolves and is absorbed through the urethra into the cavernosal bodies. This results in dilation of the cavernosal erectile tissue of the erectile chambers. See fig. 16-2. MUSE was developed by Dr. Virgil Place, a prostate cancer survivor who disliked having to give himself injections.

It has about a 66% success rate in the clinical studies. The man is instructed to void prior to using the medication. He then inserts the applicator into his penis and releases the medication. The penis is massaged and usually within 10-20 minutes, the man will achieve an erection. It has been well tolerated by most men and there have been no side effects from women with possible transfer of seminal fluid. MUSE has been effective in a certain group of patients who have been very happy with their results.

The VIVUS Company has recently re-formulated MUSE by adding a drug they call ALIBRA to make it easier to be absorbed and more efficacious. They are also developing PDE5 inhibitors for both men and women. To find out more about Vivus, go to www.vivus.com.

INJECTION THERAPY

Injection therapy was first introduced at the American Urology Association meeting in Las Vegas in 1984. Dr. Brindley was presenting a paper on how the medication, Papaverine, could be used to dilate the blood vessels in the penis and create an erection.

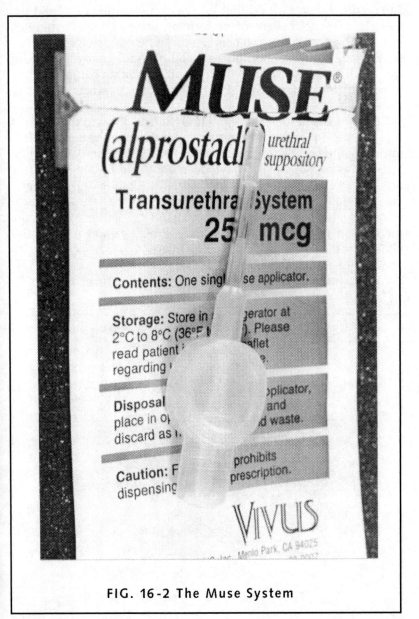

FIG. 16-2 The Muse System

Papaverine had been used in open heart surgery to dilate blood vessels which were in spasm following the bypass procedure. When Papaverine was squirted on the coronary vessels, they would dilate and allow them to function properly.

When Dr. Brindley made his presentation at the convention about Papaverine he was afraid that no one in the audience would believe him. He told them of performing an injection 45 minutes prior to the speech. At the completion of his talk, he dropped his trousers in front of 3,000 doctors and gave them absolute proof that the injections worked. There he stood, with a complete erection while the audience stared in shock. Thus, the world was introduced to penile injection therapy.

This was the first effective medical therapy. Prior to this form of therapy, the only effective treatment was through the use of penile implants and the vacuum erection device. Today there are two injection medications which have been approved by the FDA. They are Caverject, manufactured by Pharmacia-Upjohn and the medication, Edex, manufactured by Scwharz Pharma. These medications are effective in about 85% of patients. The active erectile medication in both of these drugs is Prostaglandin E. Fig. 16-3 shows the Caverject kit. An injection instruction insert comes with the Caverject kit.

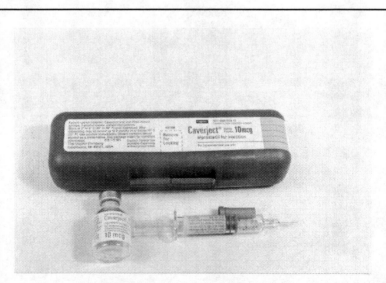

FIG. 16-3 A Caverject Kit

BI-MIX AND TRI-MIX

Occasionally, Papaverine by itself or with Regitine will be used. When the two are mixed it is called a bi-mix. Prostaglandin E1 may also be addedfor a tri-mix. This tri-mix combination usually works better than any one of them used alone. The bi-mix and tri-mix are usually much less expensive than Caverject or Edex.

PHYSIOLOGY OF THE INJECTION

Injection therapy works by relaxing the smooth muscles in the arterioles of the penis. The arteries of the penis are fairly deep, the veins are near the surface. The penis has several tubular layers or sheaths around it. As the blood flow to the penis increases, the pressure squeezes and presses the veins against the outer sheaths of the penis. The pressure closes the veins so that little of the blood can escape from the penis. This makes the penis rigid and firm.

Approximately 80% of erectile problems are associated with vascular problems. There is either not enough blood being delivered to the penile chambers, or there is too much escaping through veins which are not closed effectively. Injection therapy increases the blood flow to the penile chambers and is able to achieve good results unless there is significant vascular problems.

ADVANTAGES OF INJECTION THERAPY

Injection therapy has been a very successful mode of treatment. Between 85%-90% of men respond with good results. It has offered many men and their partners a very effective way of regaining their sexual relationship. Frequently, men will even regain their own natural erections.

Some men will have erections lasting just a few minutes and others can have the dose titrated up to allow a 30-45 minute erection. The length of time is directly related to the dose of the medication used. An infrequent problem can be an erection that lasts between 2-4 hours or more. If it lasts longer than 4 hours, he may need to go to emergency. This is called priapism. If the blood is trapped in the penis for a long period of time it can become gangrenous.

Injection therapy can be very useful in men recovering from radical prostatectomy where the nerves may have been bruised or in shock, or if the nerves were completely severed. If the nerves are still intact, the use of the injection may help in erectile recovery. Injection therapy immediately following radical prostatectomy or radiation therapy may prevent atrophy of the smooth muscle necessary for erections.

We mentioned earlier that about one third of the penis is inside the body. If a man uses a vacuum erection device (VED) to create an erection, only the part of the penis on the outside will be firm. The part of the penis inside the body may not be filled with blood. The penis will have what has been described as the "hinge effect." It may flop around from side to side and will not have the upward angle. This may not be attractive but it does not detract from the pleasure. The injection therapy causes all of the penile tissues to become engorged, even that inside the pelvic area. This makes it more like a normal erection.

DISADVANTAGES OF INJECTION THERAPY

The fear of the penile injection is what scares every man to the core when he is first informed of this form of treatment. The thought of a penile injection is totally foreign to every man. Sticking a needle into such a sensitive area is difficult for any man to accept. I have found that the man's fearful expectations are much worse than the actual injection process. Some men visualize the injection going into the glans penis. In actuality, it goes into the side of the penis and feels like a tiny pinch.

When examining a patient, I will often pinch him at the base of the penis and ask him would he be willing to trade that pinch for a 45 minute erection. Most men are willing to try an injection for diagnostic or therapeutic evaluations. We have been able to overcome the fear by using an automatic injection device. This hides the needle and automatically injects the medication with minimal discomfort. The whole process is more of a mental issue than the actual discomfort of the injection.

The injection device works so quickly that a man doesn't even realize that it has taken place. The automatic injector is spring loaded and fires when a button is depressed. The erection is usually complete within 5 to 10 minutes.

The most common side effects of injection therapy include minor bruising and discomfort. There can be possible scarring to the penile chambers. A few patients may experience an aching sensation in the erectile chambers, especially with the Caverject or Edex Prostaglandin E1.

AUTOINJECTOR

One big problem with injections is that, like most people, I (Aubrey) hate needles. I have given gallons of blood. I didn't mind the small amount of pain when I thought about the fact that I might be helping to save someone's life. But to stick a needle into my penis is something else.

Actually there is very little pain associated with the injection. But when I had the opportunity to purchase an autoinjector, I grabbed it. The autoinjector is a spring loaded device. You fill the syringe with the drug, place it in the autoinjector, then press a button and it automatically does the rest. This is a tool that can be used by diabetics or by anyone for any type of injections. The Owen Mumford Company at (770) 425-5138 manufactures several different types of auto injectors. Call them for a list of dealers. A few of the dealers are the St. Louis Medical Pharmacy at 800-950-6020, the Diabetic Express at 800-338-4656 and the Diabetic Wholesale Supply at 800-925-8299.

It is best if both the man and his partner have been involved in the diagnosis and the injection process. Frequently women feel left out of the injection therapy process. Since it affects them also, it is much better if it is explained so that they are a part of the process.

ERECTILE DYSFUNCTION PAPERS AT AUA

There were 89 papers presented on erectile dysfunction at the American Urological Association Convention in Atlanta, April 29-May 4, 2000. In addition, there were six papers presented on female sexual dysfunction.

Here are some resources on the Internet that was posted by a friend Charo Boyett:

I have listed below several URLs where more information may be found on injection therapy for ED:

Impotence FAQ
http://www.palace.net/~llama/asifaq.html
It has a section for each type of ED treatment and frequently asked questions for each.

Autoinjector source list.
Medical Center Pharmacy
http://mccpharmacy.com/trimix.html
Discussion of and explanation of different type "'mixes."

Caverject
http://www.caverject.com/

Rockwell Physicians Supplies
http://www.rockwell-physicians.com/rockwell.map?142,11

A general discussion site for injection and "mixes." With specific how-to-inject information.

Baylor ED site
http://www.urol.bcm.tmc.edu/wwwroot/erectdys.htm
Site discusses all type ED treatments. Specific info for injections. Great graphics on how-to and where-to inject.

TREATMENT WITH A PENILE PROSTHESIS

Proceeding with a penile prosthesis can be one of the most difficult steps for a patient to take. Most patients are extremely nervous, anxious and fearful about a penile implant. Many patients will not even consider an implant as a viable option in the treatment plan. Common questions are, "How can all that equipment fit into me? Will sex feel natural? Will I be able to ejaculate? Will other people know that I have an implant? Will I look natural?" These questions and many more need to be asked and answered.

Getting a penile implant is a very serious decision. The patient and his partner should never be forced into any specific type of treatment. I like patients to consider proceeding with an implant only after they have been fully educated on all of the treatment options and are completely ready emotionally and intellectually.

HOW DOES A PENILE IMPLANT WORK?

A penile implant gives rigidity to the penis. There are two erectile chambers which normally fill with blood. An implant is a cylindrical device which fills the erectile chambers and gives rigidity during the sexual act, allowing a man to once again enjoy normal sexual relations. Over 250,000 implants have been placed. Men can usually still achieve orgasm and ejaculation with an implant if they were able to do so before.

Men who become impotent following radical surgery, radiation, or cryosurgery, may find the emission of seminal fluid decreased or completely absent. However, they will still experience the sensation of orgasm. The implant works by giving penile rigidity and consists of several basic types:

Semi-Rigid Implants

These were the first implants developed. They are made of silicone and may have an internal core of a braided silver wire which helps them to be pushed downward when the prosthesis is not in use and to be placed upward when a man wants to be sexually active.

These types of implants are usually placed in the man who has arthritis and has decreased manual dexterity. They are simpler and have fewer things that can go wrong. There are fewer malfunctions of this type device that might require revision work. More physicians know how to put in these types of implant and they are easier to install.

Inflatable Penile Prosthesis

This implant was developed by Dr. Brantley Scott in 1973. Today this offers the most effective way of fixing the impotency problem. We are looking at very good success rates with the new products. Initially the inflatable penile prosthesis had many problems, but they have been re-engineered. Today, we are looking at about a 90-95% success rate at 5 years after implantation. This means that if 100 implants were placed, about 90 of them would still be functioning in 5 years.

We have stronger, better materials available today. The problem areas or weak links in the implant have been redesigned to allow a much more natural product which has seen very good patient and partner acceptance. In fact, both manufacturers of the inflatable penile prosthesis give the patient a lifetime guarantee on their products with free replacement of the implant if there should ever be a mechanical malfunction. Fig. 16-4 shows an inflatable implant from

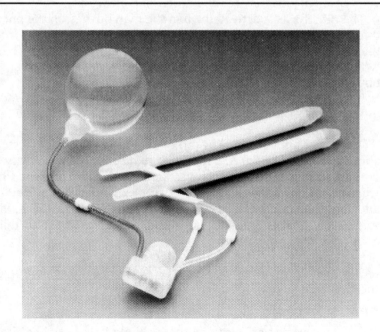

FIG. 16-4 An inflatable penile implant (Courtesy AMS)

American Medical Systems (AMS), a division of Pfizer. The AMS Company has a web site about their Penile Prosthesis Product Line: http://www.visitams.com/products/index.asp

This site has drawings and more information about all of the different penile implants.

The inflatable penile prosthesis consists of two cylinders which are implanted into the penis. A pump is placed in the scrotum, and a reservoir is placed either behind the abdominal muscles or in the scrotum. The complete device is under the skin and is not visible to the naked eye.

A man can shower at his golf, tennis, or health club without anyone being aware of his implant. These prostheses can be inserted at an outpatient surgery center or as an inpatient in the hospital. The procedure takes about one hour or less in an experienced surgeon's hands. Most men tolerate the surgery very well. I tell my patients that this procedure causes about as much discomfort as a glorified hernia procedure. The scrotal area is usually the most tender and there is a heavy feeling in that part of the body for 2-4 weeks. Most men can return to their work within 1 to 4 weeks depending on the physical demands of their job. Men who perform very physical jobs may require more time off work.

The prosthesis is activated when the man pushes on the pump through the scrotal skin. The pumping action transfers fluid from the reservoir into the penile implants in the erectile bodies. These types of devices have been very successful and seem natural for both the man and woman.

Implants may only be necessary in about 10% of patients. Most other patients can be treated medically or with a vacuum erection device (VED).

The penile implants may be rather expensive. There was a story about a man who went to a urologist to discuss the possibility of getting an implant. Since this was something that concerned his wife, he brought her along. The doctor explained the procedure and told the couple that it would cost about $10,000. The wife said, "Wow, that is an awful lot of money. We will have to think about it and let you know."

A few days later, she called the doctor and said, "About the penile implants, we have made a decision. We have decided to redo the kitchen instead."

ORAL SEX

The penis can be very clean so there should be no qualms about oral sex or fellatio. The vagina can also be very clean. A special bacteria usually lives in the vagina which converts the vaginal flu-ids to a weak acid. This acid prevents most other bacteria from invading the vagina. Women are cautioned not to use harsh mate-rials to douche because it may kill off the friendly bacteria.

Oral sex can be quite pleasurable to both men and women.

MASTURBATION

The ability for a man to have an orgasm doesn't necessarily de-pend on a firm erection. With sufficient arousal and stimulation, a man can have quite a good orgasm even without a prostate and with a limp and flaccid penis. Of course without a partial erection, it is very difficult to perform intercourse. Many women can have a good orgasm with oral and clitoral stimulation. After all, the clito-ris is a miniature penis. Some women may prefer clitoral stimula-tion rather than internal vaginal thrusting.

Some women enjoy having their "G" spot stimulated. The G spot is in the upper part of the vagina, about one inch from the vaginal opening. The G spot can be stimulated by hand, vibrator, or best of all, by a good erect penis.

The G spot is about where a prostate would be if a woman had one. In some women, the G spot is very sensitive, in others it doesn't even seem to be there.

Some women wouldn't ever consider masturbation or stimulat-ing themselves. But it may be okay if someone else does it for them. Some women can have a good orgasm by getting on top and rubbing their clitoris on the penis, even if it happens to be flaccid or soft.

Of course, if she is any kind of lady, she will reciprocate and stimulate her partner, either by hand or orally. Some men can have an orgasm if the limp penis is placed against the vagina and stimu-lated by hand.

Many men of our generation don't like to talk about masturba-tion. (The term masturbate is from the Latin *manus* for hand + *stuprare* which means to rape. So literally, when one masturbates, he or she is raping oneself by hand.) To many of us masturbation is embarrassing, shameful and sinful. Only perverts and those of weak character resort to such a wicked practice.

Many of the younger generation seem to have no shame. Many of them unabashedly admit to the evil practice of self-gratification. There are many older religious men and women who were con-vinced that if they masturbated, they would surely go to hell. To-day we know that there is nothing sick or perverted about doing something that makes you feel good. It harms no one, especially, not you. Besides, your genitals belong to you. Why should anyone tell you what you cannot do with an important part of your body?

If a person is forced to go without sex, it can cause a lot of stress build-up. Masturbation can help relieve stress and nervous energy. Reduction of stress can help improve the immune system's ability to combat illnesses. Even if you are happily married, there may be times when the wife has a headache or just doesn't feel like doing it. This should not stop you from having a bit of pleasure alone.

In speaking of masturbation, Truman Capote was quoted as saying, "The good thing is that you don't have to get dressed up for it."

We would also add that you would seldom be rejected or turned down.

Some other things to consider—you don't have to buy dinner and drinks for your date. You don't have to worry about performance or whether you are pleasing someone else. You need only worry about pleasing yourself.

Husband and wife researchers, Samuel and Cynthia Janus, surveyed 2,765 men and women about their sex habits and practices. In their book, *Janus Report on Sexual Behavior*, they reported that 47 percent of the men and 23 percent of the women admitted that they masturbate on a daily or weekly basis.

The authors didn't report as to whether any of these sinful men and women were growing hair in the palms of their hands or whether any were going blind. Other disorders that may be caused by masturbation is carpal tunnel syndrome and a related disorder called repetitive strain injury (RSI). Just kidding :-) (an internet grin). But here is an item that was reported on Dr. Dean Edell's radio show and by several news agencies. A woman filed for workman's compensation, claiming Repetitive Stress Injury (RSI) which is often the same as Carpal Tunnel Syndrome (CTS).

What is unusual about this case is that the woman worked answering telephones for a phone sex operation. She was instructed to keep the customers on line as long as possible and to be as realistic as possible. To do this she held the phone in one hand and masturbated with the other, which caused the RSI. This injury has prevented her from doing her job, so she believes that she is entitled to compensation.

This report should be an ample warning—all things in moderation—or just switch hands once in a while. ☺

Notice in the Janus Report that less than one-fourth of the women admitted that they masturbate. Again, this shows the vast difference between men and women. One reason that women are not as interested in sex as men are is because they don't produce as much testosterone as men. Most of the testosterone in men come from their testicles, but about ten percent is produced by the adrenals. Women produce adrenal testosterone also. If their testosterone level goes down, then their libido diminishes. Some women who have no sex drive may be helped by supplemental testosterone. Men have searched for some sort of aphrodisiac for eons. A little bit of testosterone might be what they are looking for.

One reason why more women don't masturbate could be that they don't know how. Some years ago in San Francisco, a women's group set up a class to teach women how to masturbate, or how to get in touch with themselves. According to reports, it was a very popular class.

A comic came up with the line that said, "When you ask a man if he masturbates, about 50 percent will admit that they do. The other 50 percent will lie about it."

Anything that you do by yourself or to yourself should be nobody's business but yours. Anything that you do to another adult or with another adult, as long as you both consent, should be nobody else's business. There should absolutely be no cause for shame, guilt or a violation of law.

There was a story of a young man who got a job on a sport fishing boat to bait the hooks for the patrons. He started work as an apprentice, but he worked very hard and within six months he became a master baiter.

Modern technology has provided us with several sex toys, accessories and devices. There are some rubber toys that have the consistency and feel of real skin. Many of these things can be a great help to both men and women. Times have changed. Some people receive sex toys for birthday presents nowadays, even those who are happily married.

The sex toys and accessories are usually hidden away in sleazy adult book stores. Many people are too embarrassed to enter one of these places.

Masturbation can never be as good as the real thing. But if you take a Playboy or Penthouse magazine to bed with you, you won't go blind or grow hair in the palm of your hand. And you won't catch any of the horrible diseases such as gonorrhea or AIDS. Or be arrested for breaking the law by paying a woman for sex.

AUDIOVISUAL SEXUAL STIMULATION

Someone once said that one good fantasy is worth a thousand realities. Visual stimulation such as X-rated tapes help many people create fantasies.

For one reason or another, some people think that pornography and sexual aids in any form should be banned and outlawed. Many states and cities do not allow adult bookstores. Pornography and some of the sexual aids are of great value in the struggle against ED. Pornographic materials should be available to any adult person. Each individual should be able make up his or her own mind. No one should decide or tell an adult person what he or she can view or do in the privacy of their own bedroom. If they are not hurting anyone, why should it be any business or concern of anyone else, especially the government?

There are several mail order companies who will discreetly ship pornographic materials to you in a plain brown wrapper. If you call them, they will send you a catalog. Here are the phone numbers and web sites of a couple of companies:

Adam and Eve at 1-800-765-2326 or www.adameve.com

Direct Video & DVD at 1-800-874-8960 or www.sexvideostore.com

If your doctor is not offering the different treatment options, find one that is. This is a very exciting time for impotent couples. Most all men can be successfully treated with one of the different therapeutic options. Again, ED is one of the few medical problems that can be successfully treated and helped in almost 100% of cases.

You can be one of the success stories.

Dr. Stephen Auerbach has an office at: 400 Newport Center Drive, Suite 501, Newport Beach, CA 92660 Tel: 714-644-7200.

INDEX